Anaphylaxis

Editor

ANNE MARIE DITTO

IMMUNOLOGY AND ALLERGY CLINICS OF NORTH AMERICA

www.immunology.theclinics.com

May 2015 • Volume 35 • Number 2

ELSEVIER

1600 John F. Kennedy Boulevard • Suite 1800 • Philadelphia, Pennsylvania, 19103-2899
http://www.theclinics.com

IMMUNOLOGY AND ALLERGY CLINICS OF NORTH AMERICA Volume 35, Number 2
May 2015 ISSN 0889-8561, ISBN-13: 978-0-323-37601-3

Editor: Jessica McCool
Developmental Editor: Stephanie Carter

Immunology and Allergy Clinics of North America (ISSN 0889–8561) is published quarterly by Elsevier Inc., 360 Park Avenue South, New York, NY 10010-1710. Months of issue are February, May, August, and November. Periodicals postage paid at New York, NY and additional mailing offices. Subscription prices are $320.00 per year for US individuals, $454.00 per year for US institutions, $150.00 per year for US students and residents, $395.00 per year for Canadian individuals, $220.00 per year for Canadian students, $577.00 per year for Canadian institutions, $445.00 per year for international individuals, $577.00 per year for international institutions, $220.00 per year for international students. To receive student/resident rate, orders must be accompanied by name of affiliated institution, date of term, and the *signature* of program/residency coordinator on institution letterhead. Orders will be billed at individual rate until proof of status is received. Foreign air speed delivery is included in all *Clinics* subscription prices. All prices are subject to change without notice. **POSTMASTER**: Send address changes to *Immunology and Allergy Clinics of North America*, Elsevier Health Sciences Division, Subscription Customer Service, 3251 Riverport Lane, Maryland Heights, MO 63043. **Customer Service: 1-800-654-2452 (U.S. and Canada); 314-447-8871 (outside U.S. and Canada). Fax: 314-447-8029. E-mail: journalscustomerservice-usa@elsevier.com (for print support); journalsonlinesupport-usa@elsevier.com (for online support).**

Reprints. For copies of 100 or more, of articles in this publication, please contact the Commercial Reprints Department, Elsevier Inc., 360 Park Avenue South, New York, New York 10010-1710. Tel. 212-633-3874, Fax: 212-633-3820, E-mail: reprints@elsevier.com.

Immunology and Allergy Clinics of North America is covered in MEDLINE/PubMed (Index Medicus), Current Contents/Life Sciences, Science Citation Index, ISI/BIOMED, Chemical Abstracts, and EMBASE/Excerpta Medica.

Contributors

EDITOR

ANNE MARIE DITTO, MD
Associate Professor of Medicine, Division of Allergy-Immunology, Department of Medicine, Northwestern University Feinberg School of Medicine, Chicago, Illinois

AUTHORS

CEM AKIN, MD, PhD
Director, Mastocytosis Center, Brigham and Women's Hospital; Associate Professor of Medicine, Harvard Medical School, Boston, Massachusetts

JONATHAN A. BERNSTEIN, MD
Division of Immunology, Allergy and Rheumatology, Department of Medicine, University of Cincinnati College of Medicine; Bernstein Clinical Research Center, Cincinnati, Ohio

MARIANA C. CASTELLS, MD, PhD
Director, Allergy Immunology Training Program; Director, Drug Hypersensitivity and Desensitization Center; Associate Director, Mastocytosis Center, Brigham and Women's Hospital; Associate Professor of Medicine, Harvard Medical School, Boston, Massachusetts

SCOTT P. COMMINS, MD, PhD
Associate Professor of Medicine, Asthma and Allergic Diseases Center, University of Virginia Health System, Charlottesville, Virginia

ANNA M. FELDWEG, MD
Clinical Instructor in Medicine, Division of Rheumatology, Immunology, and Allergy, Brigham and Women's Hospital, Harvard Medical School, Boston, Massachusetts

NANA FENNY, MD, MPH
Allergy and Immunology Fellow, Division of Allergy and Immunology, Department of Medicine, Northwestern University Feinberg School of Medicine, Chicago, Illinois

ANNA B. FISHBEIN, MD, MSCI
Attending Physician, Allergy/Immunology; Assistant Professor of Pediatrics, Ann & Robert H Lurie Children's Hospital of Chicago, Chicago, Illinois

DAVID B.K. GOLDEN, MD
Associate Professor of Medicine, Johns Hopkins University, Baltimore, Maryland

LESLIE C. GRAMMER, MD
Professor of Medicine, Division of Allergy and Immunology, Department of Medicine, Northwestern University Feinberg School of Medicine, Chicago, Illinois

PAUL A. GREENBERGER, MD
Professor of Medicine, Division of Allergy and Immunology, Department of Medicine, Northwestern University Feinberg School of Medicine, Chicago, Illinois

JENNIFER A. KANNAN, MD
Division of Immunology, Allergy and Rheumatology, Department of Medicine, University of Cincinnati College of Medicine, Cincinnati, Ohio

ANN M. KEMP, RPh, MD, FAAFP
Clinical Associate Professor of Pharmacy Practice; Associate Professor, Department of Family Medicine, The University of Mississippi Medical Center, Jackson, Mississippi

STEPHEN F. KEMP, MD
Professor of Medicine and Pediatrics, Division of Clinical Immunology and Allergy, Department of Medicine, The University of Mississippi Medical Center, Jackson, Mississippi

DAVID A. KHAN, MD
Professor of Medicine and Pediatrics, Division of Allergy and Immunology, Department of Internal Medicine, University of Texas Southwestern Medical Center, Dallas, Texas

MERIN KURUVILLA, MD
Park City Allergy and Asthma, Dallas, Texas

MELANIE M. MAKHIJA, MD, MSc
Attending Physician, Allergy/Immunology; Assistant Professor of Pediatrics, Ann & Robert H Lurie Children's Hospital of Chicago, Chicago, Illinois

LINDSEY E. MOORE, DO
Fellow, Allergy and Immunology, Division of Clinical Immunology and Allergy, Department of Medicine, The University of Mississippi Medical Center, Jackson, Mississippi

THOMAS A.E. PLATTS-MILLS, MD, PhD, FRS
Professor of Medicine, Asthma and Allergic Diseases Center, University of Virginia Health System, Charlottesville, Virginia

JACQUELINE A. PONGRACIC, MD
Division Head, Allergy/Immunology; Professor of Pediatrics and Medicine, Ann & Robert H Lurie Children's Hospital of Chicago, Chicago, Illinois

ALEXANDER J. SCHUYLER, BS, BA
Graduate Student, Asthma and Allergic Diseases Center, University of Virginia Health System, Charlottesville, Virginia

ANUBHA TRIPATHI, MD
Assistant Professor of Medicine, Asthma and Allergic Diseases Center, University of Virginia Health System, Charlottesville, Virginia

Contents

reactions at first exposure. Severe hypersensitivity can preclude first-line therapy. Tryptase level at the time of a reaction is a useful diagnostic tool. Skin testing provides a specific diagnosis. Newer tests are promising diagnostic tools to help identify patients at risk before first exposure. Safe management includes rapid drug desensitization. This review provides information regarding the scope of hypersensitivity and anaphylactic reactions induced by chemotherapy and biological drugs, as well as diagnosis, management, and treatment options.

Nana Fenny and Leslie C. Grammer

Idiopathic anaphylaxis is a diagnosis of exclusion after other causes have been thoroughly evaluated and excluded. The pathogenesis of idiopathic anaphylaxis remains uncertain, although increased numbers of activated lymphocytes and circulating histamine-releasing factors have been implicated. Signs and symptoms of patients diagnosed with idiopathic anaphylaxis are indistinguishable from the manifestations of other forms of anaphylaxis. Treatment regimens are implemented based on the frequency and severity of patient symptoms and generally include the use of epinephrine autoinjectors, antihistamines, and steroids. The prognosis of idiopathic anaphylaxis is generally favorable with well-established treatment regimens and effective patient education.

Lindsey E. Moore, Ann M. Kemp, and Stephen F. Kemp

Anaphylaxis is an acute and potentially lethal multisystem allergic reaction that occurs in a variety of clinical scenarios and is almost unavoidable. Immunologic reactions to medications, foods, and insect stings cause most episodes, but virtually any substance capable of inducing systemic degranulation of mast cells and basophils can produce anaphylaxis. All health care professionals must be able to recognize anaphylaxis promptly, be prepared to treat it appropriately, and be able to provide preventive recommendations. Similarly, at-risk individuals must be prepared to self-treat anaphylaxis promptly if prevention fails.

Paul A. Greenberger

Anaphylaxis implies a risk of death even in patients whose prior episodes have been considered mild and managed easily. Anaphylaxis occurs in all age groups, from infants to the elderly, but most deaths occur in adults. Factors or circumstances associated with near-fatal or fatal anaphylaxis are reviewed from the following 10 perspectives: accidents and mishaps, adulterated products, age, allergens, atopy, comorbidities, Munchausen syndrome or contrived anaphylaxis, patient factors, route of administration, and treatment-related issues. There are no absolute contraindications to self-injectable epinephrine, and epinephrine can be administered for anaphylaxis to elderly patients or to those patients receiving beta-adrenergic blockers.

viii *Anaphylaxis*

IMMUNOLOGY AND ALLERGY
CLINICS OF NORTH AMERICA

FORTHCOMING ISSUES

August 2015
Eosinophil-Associated Disorders
Amy D. Klion and
Princess Ogbogu, *Editors*

November 2015
Primary Immunodeficiency Disorders
Anthony Montanaro, *Editor*

February 2016
Aeroallergen and Food Immunotherapy
Linda Cox and Anna Nowak-Wegrzyn,
Editors

RECENT ISSUES

February 2015
Pediatric Allergy
Robert Wood, Pamela Frischmeyer-
Guerrerio, and Corinne Keet, *Editors*

November 2014
Obesity and Asthma
Anurag Agrawal, *Editor*

August 2014
Drug Hypersensitivity
Pascal Demoly, *Editor*

ISSUE OF RELATED INTEREST

Emergency Medicine Clinics, November 2014 (Vol. 32, Issue 4)
Critical Care Emergencies
Evie Marcolini and Haney Mallemat, *Editors*
http://www.emed.theclinics.com/

NOW AVAILABLE FOR YOUR iPhone and iPad

Preface
Anaphylaxis

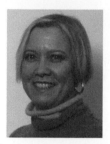

Anne Marie Ditto, MD
Editor

It has been more than a century since Portier and Richet first described anaphylaxis—a severe, potentially life-threatening IgE-mediated allergic reaction. This term is now used to describe all clinically similar reactions, underscoring the life-threatening severity, no matter the cause. The World Allergy Organization has proposed that the term *anaphylactoid* be replaced by *nonimmunologic anaphylaxis*, while the term *immunologic anaphylaxis* be used to describe IgE-mediated and other immunologic reactions.

This issue of *Immunology and Allergy Clinics of North America* is aimed at providing insight into new discoveries, as well as known causes, prevention, and treatment of anaphylaxis. Newer topics include the following: successful desensitization protocols for non-IgE-mediated reactions; anaphylaxis with first exposure due to sensitization to a common carbohydrate through tick bites; the increasing role that food plays in (possibly) all types of exercise-induced anaphylaxis; and mast cell disorders, including the spectrum of mast cell activation syndrome. Other articles in this issue are dedicated to the major causes of anaphylaxis—food, venom, and drugs (with perioperative anaphylaxis addressed separately)—idiopathic anaphylaxis, treatment of anaphylaxis, and factors that contribute to poor outcomes. Each article is authored by experts, well known in the field of Allergy-Immunology, whose contributions have helped further the knowledge and understanding of anaphylaxis.

Anne Marie Ditto, MD
Division of Allergy-Immunology
Department of Medicine
Northwestern University Feinberg School of Medicine
211 East Ontario, Room 1009
Chicago, IL 60611, USA

E-mail address:
amditto@northwestern.edu

http://dx.doi.org/10.1016/j.iac.2015.01.012
0889-8561/15/$ – see front matter © 2015 Published by Elsevier Inc.
immunology.theclinics.com

Anaphylaxis to Food

Anna B. Fishbein, MD, MSCI, Melanie M. Makhija, MD, MSc,
Jacqueline A. Pongracic, MD*

KEYWORDS

- Food-induced anaphylaxis • Dietary avoidance • Emergency preparedness
- Epinephrine autoinjectors

KEY POINTS

- Anaphylaxis to food is a growing personal and public health concern.
- Comorbid asthma, delayed administration of epinephrine, and age (teens and young adults) are factors associated with increased risk of fatal and near-fatal reactions.
- Cofactors such as exercise or concurrent ingestion of alcohol, aspirin, or nonsteroidal anti-inflammatory medications should be considered in the evaluation of patients with food-induced anaphylaxis.
- Health care providers should prescribe epinephrine autoinjectors, provide written emergency action plans, and review their appropriate use on an ongoing basis.

INTRODUCTION

Anaphylaxis related to foods is of growing concern, not only for individuals who must maintain constant vigilance against accidental exposures and manage uncertainty about severity of future reactions but also for society at large, given the prominent role of food in social settings and the direct and downstream economic costs related to health care utilization. This article is intended to provide the reader with a clinically oriented review of the epidemiology, risk factors, allergens, diagnosis, and management of food-induced anaphylaxis.

EPIDEMIOLOGY

Most epidemiologic studies of food-induced anaphylaxis have focused on analysis of emergency department visits and hospitalizations. Investigative approaches targeting discharge codes and using consensus reports and expert review for diagnosis have been used to overcome challenges related to the variable presentation of anaphylaxis

The authors have nothing to disclose.
Allergy/Immunology, Ann & Robert H Lurie Children's Hospital of Chicago, 225 East Chicago Avenue #60, Chicago, IL 60611, USA
* Corresponding author.
E-mail address: jpongracic@luriechildrens.org

Immunol Allergy Clin N Am 35 (2015) 231–245
http://dx.doi.org/10.1016/j.iac.2015.01.003
0889-8561/15/$ – see front matter © 2015 Elsevier Inc. All rights reserved.

and inconsistencies in diagnosis. In the United States, a multicenter study estimated that nearly one-half million emergency department visits for food-induced anaphylaxis occurred between the years 2001 and 2005.[1] A time trend analysis of 2001 to 2009 US data showed that the rate of emergency department visits was stable overall and stable among children, with a decrease in adults.[2] This study also calculated that, on average, an emergency department visit for food-induced anaphylaxis occurred every 5 minutes in the United States. Although the incidence of anaphylaxis of all causes has been reported to be increasing in westernized countries, this phenomenon seems to be most prominent in young children under 5 years of age, for whom food is the most common trigger.[3]

Researchers have used other methods to study the epidemiology of food allergy and food-induced anaphylaxis. For example, geographic variations in epinephrine autoinjector prescription rates in the United States and Australia have been studied as a proxy for food allergy. Significantly higher prescription rates have been found in less sunny regions of both countries.[4,5] Of note, the Australian study also revealed that hospital anaphylaxis admission rates were significantly higher in areas having less sunlight.[5] A study of 24 pediatric hospitals in the United States found that the incidence of food-induced anaphylaxis was almost double in the north compared with the south (0.31 vs 0.17 per 1000 encounters; relative risk, 1.81; 95% confidence interval, 1.66–1.98; $P<.001$).[6] A nationally representative study of US emergency department data comparing visits for allergic reactions related to foods also found similar geographic differences.[7] Taken together, these findings have led to speculation that sunlight/vitamin D status may play an etiologic role in food allergy and perhaps its severity. More research is needed to answer this important question.

Given the risk of fatality from food allergy, investigators have also looked at trends and patterns in mortality. From 1999 to 2010, food-related causes were relatively uncommon (6.7%) as compared with medication (58.8%) and venom causes (15.2%) in a study of US mortality data from the National Center for Health Statistics.[8] Age, African American race, and male gender were significantly associated with fatal food-induced anaphylaxis. Of note, the overall rate of US mortality did not increase over the 12-year period and was similar to that reported in Australia, but the rate of fatal anaphylaxis to foods did increase among male African Americans as compared with whites and Hispanic subjects. Interestingly, the study did not find any geographic differences. Fatalities from food-induced anaphylaxis have similarly remained stable in Australia.[3]

RISK FACTORS

Risk factors for food-induced anaphylaxis are largely poorly understood. Attempts to predict severe reactions focused on easily obtainable data, such as age, gender, comorbid asthma and allergic diseases, prior food reactions, skin test, and allergen-specific immunoglobulin (sIgE), have been largely disappointing. Spontaneous basophil activation, which is not yet commercially available, has been found to be higher in children with more severe milk-induced reactions.[9]

To date, the factors that have been most commonly associated with fatality include peanut or tree nut allergy, presence of asthma (particularly severe or poorly controlled asthma), lack of access to epinephrine, failure to administer epinephrine promptly, upright (rather than supine) position during a reaction involving the cardiovascular system, and age, with teenagers and young adults at highest risk.[10–13] Whether this last association is related to age-associated risk-taking behavior or other factors is unclear.

For some individuals, exercise is a necessary cofactor, as is seen in food-dependent, exercise-induced, anaphylaxis (FDEIAn). Whether a food allergen is ingested alone or in association with other foods or medications has also been proposed to contribute to the development of anaphylaxis. For example, a small study of patients with apple-induced anaphylaxis suggested that fasting was associated with the development of symptoms and proposed rapid pepsin-digestion and absorption as possible mechanisms.[14] There is also evidence that ingestion of alcohol, aspirin, and nonsteroidal anti-inflammatory medications in association with food allergen seems to escalate absorption, leading to more severe reactions.[15] More research in larger populations is needed to understand the relative contribution of these factors to the onset and severity of food-induced anaphylaxis.

ALLERGENS

Any food may cause anaphylaxis, but certain foods are more commonly associated with severe reactions. Peanut, tree nuts, and seafood represent the most frequent food triggers of anaphylaxis among children and adults. For young children, cow milk and egg are very common culprits. In fact, cow milk has been reported to account for up to 13% of fatal food-induced anaphylaxis.[12] Although 75% of children with cow milk allergy tolerate milk in baked forms, children who are reactive to baked milk have been found to have a higher risk of severe and protracted anaphylaxis requiring epinephrine.[16]

Lipid transfer protein (LTP) is a pan-allergen found in plants that is resistant to heat and pepsin digestion. LTP is found in many fruits and vegetables, some grains, as well as peanut and tree nuts. It is known to be a common cause of food allergy, most often associated with peach ingestion, in adults residing in Mediterranean areas.[17] Of note, LTP is different from the heat-labile allergens, such as profilins and allergens from the PR-10 family, which are involved in the food-pollen syndrome. Recent reports from Italy have implicated LTP as a common cause of food-induced anaphylaxis.[18] Severe LTP-induced reactions are seen in individuals who do not have cosensitization to the labile allergens of the food-pollen syndrome; co-sensitization to these allergens has been reported to decrease the severity of LTP reactions.[18] LTP has also been proposed to be the most frequent cause of FDEIAn in Italy. Sensitization to Pru p 3 (peach LTP) was noted in 78% of 82 patients with FDEIAn for whom tomato, cereals, and peanut, foods that are known to contain LTP, were the most commonly suspected food triggers.[19]

Nearly a decade ago, severe, sometimes fatal anaphylactic reactions were being seen in association with the first infusion of cetuximab, a chimeric epidermal growth factor receptor inhibitor that was being used to treat cancer. These individuals, who resided in areas associated with high prevalence of Rocky Mountain spotted fever, were found to have preexisting IgE to galactose-α-1,3-galactose (α-gal), which is present on the heavy chain of cetuximab. Subsequent investigation found that bites from the lone star tick accounted for IgE to α-gal. Interestingly, α-gal is also a major blood group substance of nonprimate mammals. Some of the affected patients reported that their reactions began more than 3 hours after eating red meat. Since then, beef, pork, and lamb have been shown to contain the α-gal allergen and to induce such delayed anaphylaxis. Allergen-sIgE to α-gal has been demonstrated in adults and more recently in children with this entity.[20,21]

DIAGNOSIS

In general, the diagnosis of IgE-mediated food allergy is established by history and further supported by documentation of the presence of sIgE to the suspected food. Physical examination is usually not helpful, unless the examination is performed during an acute reaction. However, findings of other allergic diseases may help guide one toward the diagnosis. Manifestations of anaphylaxis generally occur within minutes and up to 2 hours of ingestion of a culprit food.[22] Food-associated biphasic anaphylactic reactions are characterized by an initial reaction followed by recurrence of symptoms within 2 to 24 hours after original ingestion; biphasic reactions are infrequent, occurring in only ~2% of oral food challenges.[23,24] The diagnosis of anaphylaxis to a food allergen requires diagnostic criteria for anaphylaxis. Briefly, anaphylaxis is generally defined by the involvement of 2 or more organ systems: cutaneous, respiratory, gastrointestinal, and/or cardiovascular. Symptoms may initially present as subtle as a few hives or 1 episode of emesis, and extreme caution should be taken to monitor for progression of symptoms to include other organ systems. Severe anaphylaxis can occur in the absence of cutaneous symptoms, which can cause a delay in recognition and treatment of symptoms. Vigilance to recognize subtle symptoms of anaphylaxis, such as cough or voice changes, is crucial in making the diagnosis.

Determining the culprit food in the case of anaphylaxis can be difficult, especially if multiple foods were consumed. For this reason, obtaining a history as soon as possible regarding timing of the reaction and gathering ingredient information is crucial to identifying the culprit food. Although double-blind food challenge to an implicated food is the gold standard in diagnosing food allergy, it is often unnecessary in the setting of convincing history, particularly in the case of severe reactions and supportive diagnostic testing. History should direct the choice of allergens for skin-prick and/or in vitro testing.

Differential Diagnosis

A thorough evaluation should take into consideration the many causes discussed in this issue. Close association between the time of ingestion and onset of reaction helps to narrow the differential diagnosis toward food. Most non-IgE-mediated food reactions do not induce anaphylaxis, except for specific cases such as Scombroid poisoning, in which manifestations are often localized to the skin and gastrointestinal tract but rarely may affect the respiratory and cardiovascular systems. Food protein-induced enterocolitis syndrome (FPIES) reactions may induce significant vomiting and/or diarrhea, resulting in hypovolemia and subsequent hypotension, which may be confused with anaphylaxis. Timing of FPIES reactions tends to be more delayed than IgE-mediated reactions, generally occurring 1 to 5 hours after ingestion of the offending food.[25]

Testing Options

The initial approach to food allergy testing standardly involves either skin testing (prick or puncture) or serum sIgE testing for implicated allergens. Other modalities are becoming standardized, such as component-resolved diagnostics and the basophil activation test (BAT), both of which may also predict severity of reactions. Aside from these tests, there are currently no other assays to predict severity of reactions to food allergens. Intradermal testing to foods is never recommended given the lack of correlation with clinical reactivity and the risk of untoward reactions.[26]

Skin Testing

Skin prick or puncture testing is performed using purified allergen extracts or fresh foods along with positive and negative controls. Measurement of the resultant wheal and flare is performed, and a positive result is generally considered to be a wheal size at least 3 mm larger than the negative control. In general, skin testing has high sensitivity and low specificity. Several research studies have assessed the positive and negative predictive value of skin testing in predicting food allergy to the most common food allergens (**Tables 1** and **2**). A list of these values for various allergens, compiled from a variety of published articles, is summarized in **Tables 1** and **2**. In applying these findings to a broader population, one should consider the demographics of the research population, such as degree of atopy (for example, presence or absence of atopic dermatitis) and country of recruitment. Skin prick testing can give false negative results in children less than 4 to 6 months of age or if histamine blocking medications are being taken.[26]

Serum Allergen-Specific Immunoglobulin E Testing

Serum sIgE testing measures circulating sIgE using fluorescence enzyme immunoassay. Previously, sIgE testing was performed using radioallergosorbent test technology, which has been improved with ELISAs, such as ImmunoCAP (Phadia, Uppsala, Sweden) and IMMULITE (Siemens Healthcare Diagnostics, Tarrytown, NY, USA) systems. Some studies suggest similar results between these testing modalities,[27] while others suggest slightly higher sIgE results in the Immulite system.[28] Most research studies have used the ImmunoCAP system, because it has been available for a long time. The positive and negative predictive values of sIgE testing are summarized in **Tables 1** and **2**.

Panels of food allergen testing are not recommended, because they can result in false positive testing and unnecessary dietary restriction.[22] In fact, one study found that 80% of children sensitized to peanut as determined by skin test and sIgE were not actually clinically reactive.[29] Careful history and determination of pretest probability of a reaction are crucial to the interpretation of food allergen testing. Although false negative tests are uncommon, it is important to remember that in the setting of a convincing history, negative in vitro testing does not necessarily eliminate the possibility of food allergy.

Component-Resolved Diagnostics

Component testing measures sIgE to specific allergen epitopes in serum via automated microarray. This test serves as another tool to predict the likelihood of food allergy. It can also be helpful in indicating when a severe reaction, such as anaphylaxis, is more likely to

Table 1
The positive predictive value of sensitization in predicting food allergy

	sIgE ≥0.35 kU/L,[a] % (Reference)	Skin Prick Test ≥3 mm, % (Reference)
Milk	35[68]–~60[69,70]	~65[70]
Egg	30[68]–~90[70,71]	~90[70,71]
Peanut	40[72]	75[73]
Tree nuts	30–40[72,74]	n/a
Fish	~50[70]	~75[70]
Shellfish	42[75]	30[75]–55[76]
Wheat	~15[68,70]	35[70]
Soy	15[68]–21[70]	35[70]
Sesame	10–22[72,77]	31[77]

Abbreviation: n/a, not available.
[a] Immunocap and IMMULITE systems are highly correlated; results of sIgE are considered equivalent for purposes of this review.

Table 2
95% or greater positive predictive value in predicting food allergy

	sIgE kU/L ≥95% PPV (Reference)	Skin Prick Test, mm Wheal ≥95% PPV (Reference)
Milk	15–32[78]–90[68,a]	8[79]
Egg	1.7[80]–6[78]–13[68]	4[80]–7[79]
Baked egg	50[80,a,b]	11[80,a,b]
Peanut	13[72]–34[80]–>100[81]	8[80]–16[73]
Tree nuts	15–>100[72]	8[82]
Fish	20[70]	n/a
Shellfish	n/a	~20[76]
Wheat	50[68,c]–100[70]	n/a
Soy	65[70,a]≥100[68,c]	n/a
Sesame	17.5–50[a,77,80]	8–23[77,80]

Abbreviations: n/a, not available; PPV, positive predictive value.
[a] 80%–95% PPV.
[b] sIgE or skin prick testing to egg/egg white (not baked).
[c] 30–50% PPV.

occur. In general, allergy to multiple epitopes is considered indicative of higher severity and persistent allergy. Peanut is the most extensively studied allergen with regards to component testing. Component testing to peanut is used clinically as an adjunct to sIgE testing to whole peanut. Specifically, it can be helpful in providing more accurate diagnostic information in children who have never reacted to peanut, but have a high peanut sIgE level or who have relatively low levels but do not meet typically used criteria of 2 kU/L or less for food challenge. It has been suggested that positive component testing to Ara h2 is more sensitive and specific than sIgE to whole peanut; sIgE to AraH2 has 60% to 100% sensitivity and 60% to 90% specificity in predicting reactivity.[30] A recent article purports potential strategies for the use of peanut component testing in algorithms to reduce the need for food challenges.[31] In addition, the presence of sIgE to Ara h1-3 has been popularized as the most likely profile to indicate anaphylaxis, with Ara h9 being a more moderate risk, and Ara h8 or Ara h5 indicating the lowest risk of anaphylaxis.[32,33] However, this data to predict anaphylaxis are generated from different geographic populations for whom sensitization patterns to peanut differ, making this data difficult to broadly apply.[34,35] Another role of component testing is to differentiate patients with high sIgE who are not truly reactive, such as in those with hazelnut (+Cor a1) or peanut (+Ara h 8) sIgE and sIgE to Bet v1, indicating sensitization causing food-pollen syndrome due to cross-reactive antigens, but not true food allergy.[36]

Basophil Activation Test

BAT involves flow cytometry to detect upregulation of cell surface markers on the basophil (such as CD63) after in vitro antigen stimulation of blood. Although this test is not standardized or routinely used in North America, a recent study suggests that BAT is more accurate than skin testing, as well as sIgE and even component testing in predicting peanut allergy.[37] The current opinion is that this test might offer a way to distinguish patients who have developed tolerance to a food allergen.[9,38]

Food Challenge

A food challenge to the implicated food or foods may be indicated to elucidate the cause of anaphylaxis if other testing produces unclear results. The risk-benefit ratio must be weighed carefully in the decision to perform a food challenge when the history is that of severe anaphylaxis. Food challenges in the clinical setting are often performed as open unblinded challenges to a single food; double-blind food challenges require more labor and time. In the setting of a history of anaphylaxis, there is a risk for anaphylaxis to a food challenge, so this procedure should be done cautiously under close medical supervision in which trained personnel and emergency equipment are available to handle an anaphylactic reaction.

TREATMENT AND PREVENTION
Acute Reactions

There are currently no approved therapies to prevent IgE-mediated reactions to foods. Avoidance of allergenic foods and emergency management of acute reactions are the mainstays of treatment. Consensus guidelines for the diagnosis and management of anaphylaxis have been published.[39–41] Treatment of acute reactions to foods may be guided by the severity of the reaction, taking into account the severity of prior reactions. Severe reactions including anaphylaxis or reactions involving cardiovascular and/or respiratory symptoms require treatment with intramuscular injection of epinephrine. Aqueous epinephrine, 1:1000 dilution (1 mg/mL), 0.2–0.5 mL (0.01 mg/kg in children, max. 0.3 mg dosage; 0.3 mg–0.5 mg for adults), should be injected intramuscularly in the lateral aspect of the thigh every 5 min, as necessary, to control symptoms and increase blood pressure.[41] Epinephrine is the first-line medication for treatment of anaphylaxis. As previously noted, delay in use of epinephrine has been associated with fatal anaphylaxis.[13] A survey of 7822 caregivers and medical personnel suggests that anaphylaxis is underrecognized and epinephrine is underutilized by both groups, especially in patients who do not have skin symptoms.[42] As mentioned previously, lack of skin symptoms is a risk factor for death or near death from anaphylaxis. A review of a European anaphylaxis registry of 2000 patients who had severe anaphylactic reactions found that only 13% received epinephrine, whereas 50% received antihistamines and 51% received corticosteroids.[43]

As stated above, if symptoms persist, repeat intramuscular epinephrine doses may be given every 5 minutes. A survey of food allergic families revealed that 13% of patients who were given epinephrine for food-induced anaphylaxis required a second dose of epinephrine and 6% needed a third dose.[44] Patients in this report who required additional doses of epinephrine were more likely to have asthma.

After administration of intramuscular epinephrine for food-induced anaphylaxis, the emergency response team (eg, 911) should be called. Additional, adjunctive medications may be given, such as H1 antagonists (ie, diphenhydramine 1–2 mg/kg or 25–50 mg per dose). Although antihistamines alone are often used for mild reactions including isolated skin symptoms and mild gastrointestinal symptoms, antihistamines will not prevent the progression of a reaction and will not reverse airway obstruction or hypotension.[41] If the patient is wheezing, short of breath, or coughing, an inhaled bronchodilator (eg, albuterol MDI 2–6 puffs or nebulized, 2.5–5 mg in 3 mL saline) may be used. Often H2 antagonists are also administered, because there is some evidence that diphenhydramine and ranitidine together are better than diphenhydramine alone.[41] The patient should be placed in a supine or recumbent position with their legs elevated to increase central perfusion especially if dizziness or hypotension is present.[11] Oxygen should be given to the patient and, if necessary, an airway should be established. If the patient is not responding well to medications, intravenous fluids should be administered rapidly, especially in the setting of hypotension to help replenish intravascular volume as massive fluid shifts occur in anaphylaxis.[45]

Corticosteroids should never be given as first-line therapy in place of epinephrine; however, prednisone 1 to 2 mg/kg/d for 2 to 3 days is often prescribed as adjunctive therapy to prevent recurrence of symptoms or biphasic reactions. The evidence supporting the use of corticosteroids in anaphylaxis is limited.[41]

Biphasic reactions are relatively infrequent in food-induced anaphylaxis.[23,24] However, it is important to be aware that delayed reactions can occur and may be as severe as immediate reactions. Because of this, the current recommendations found in the National Institute of Allergy and Infectious Diseases *Guidelines for the Diagnosis and Management of Food Allergy in the United States* include observation of the patient in a medical setting for 4 to 6 hours following a reaction and sending the patient home with an autoinjectable epinephrine prescription and an emergency action plan.[45] After the acute reaction resolves, the patient should be assessed by an allergist-immunologist for further diagnosis, treatment, and prevention counseling.[41]

In addition to instructions on administration of emergency medications, emergency action plans are an important component of patient education. Education of food allergic individuals and their caregivers should include how to recognize the signs and symptoms of anaphylaxis and how to treat them appropriately when they occur. The patient or family should be given an action plan and it should be reviewed regularly at visits with an allergist or other health care provider. Food-allergic individuals should also be given prescriptions for autoinjectable epinephrine and instructed on its proper use. A recent study that assessed skin-to-bone depth (STBD) by ultrasound in children who weigh less than 15 kg found that approximately 19% of those weighing 10 to 14.9 kg and 60% of those less than 10 kg had a maximum STBD less than 12.7 mm.[46] The length of the needle for name-brand low-dose epinephrine autoinjectors (ie, Epipen Jr and Auvi-Q 0.15 mg) is 12.7 mm, thus putting these children at risk of having epinephrine injected into bone; therefore, caution must be exercised in prescribing epinephrine to very small children.

Prevention

Strict avoidance of known allergenic foods is recommended. Prevention of reactions involves significant patient and caregiver education about the food and its avoidance, including label reading, school education, eating outside the home, and possibilities of cross-contamination. Unfortunately, despite these measures, accidental exposures do occur. A prospective observational study of 512 infants with likely milk or egg allergy revealed that reactions occurred in 71.7% subjects with 52.5% reporting more than one reaction over a 36-month period.[47] Most reactions were due to accidental ingestions, label-reading errors, and cross-contamination. In 50.6% of reactions, someone other than the child's parents provided the eliciting food. Of 11.4% of reactions that were severe, only 29.9% were treated with epinephrine.[47] A Canadian study of peanut allergic children revealed an annual incidence rate of accidental exposures of 12.5%, with only 21% of moderate and severe reactions being treated with epinephrine.[48]

In some cases, patients may have a false sense of security when the culprit food allergen is identified. For example, the patient may feel avoidance of the allergen in question is under their complete control so they do not carry their autoinjectable epinephrine all of the time. A survey by Kemp and colleagues[49] found that only 47% of patients who had an identified allergen and who were prescribed epinephrine had their autoinjector with them at the time of reaction, whereas 89% of patients who had a diagnosis of idiopathic anaphylaxis had their autoinjector with them at the time of reaction. Label reading is cumbersome and food-labeling laws vary by country. The US Food Allergen Labeling and Consumer Protection Act mandates labeling in lay terms for all foods manufactured in this country. The 8 most common allergenic foods (milk, egg, peanut, tree nuts, wheat, soy, fish, and crustacean shellfish) must be listed when they are ingredients in a packaged food. The law does not apply to packaged fresh meat, poultry, egg products, or alcohol. Other allergens may not be listed clearly, and patients should be advised to call the manufacturer to clarify ingredients if necessary. Potential cross-contact must also be considered with packaged foods. Cross-contact may be reported using advisory phrases such as "processed in or manufactured in a facility with," "may contain," or "manufactured on shared equipment with." This type of voluntarily reporting by the manufacturers is not mandated by law. Patients should be advised to read labels each time they purchase a food product because ingredients may change over time. A US survey of supermarket products found that 17% of packaged products in 24 categories contained an advisory label for food allergens: 38% had "may contain"; 33% had "shared/same equipment"; and 29% had "shared facility" advisory labels.[50] As many as 40% to 54% of products examined in this study in categories including cookies, chocolate, and baking mixes had advisory labels. There is a relatively low rate of actual cross-contamination in foods with advisory labels with a recent study of products with peanut advisory labeling showing that only 8.6% of food products with peanut advisory labels contained detectable levels of peanut.[51]

Safety outside the home or away from the care of parents is a significant source of anxiety to families. Careful advanced planning and education are crucial. Always having emergency medications on hand and an emergency plan ready are critical steps for emergency management of accidental reactions. Wearing medical identification jewelry is also helpful. When eating in restaurants, vigilance must be maintained by discussing the allergy with wait staff or using written "chef cards" explaining the severity of the allergy and informing about cross-contamination.[52]

Reducing risk in the school setting is vital. Reactions from accidental ingestion at school have been reported to occur in 16% to 18% of children with food allergies.[53,54] In addition, 25% of anaphylactic episodes that occurred at school happened in children who had no previous history of food allergy.[53,55] Safety while at school includes the provision of an emergency action plan identifying allergens, explaining the manifestations and symptoms of allergic reactions and outlining a treatment plan including emergency medication and the doses recommended. The child's family is responsible for providing emergency medications, including autoinjectable epinephrine and additional medications if necessary. The school is responsible for ensuring that staff members are both adequately trained on management of the student's allergies and available at all times. A 504 Plan or individualized education program may be helpful to outline specific, mutually agreeable measures to keep the child safe at school. Safety at school also includes ensuring that the child is not being bullied because of his or her allergies. A survey of 251 families of food-allergic children found that 45.4% of kids indicated that they had been bullied; 31.5% reported bullying specifically because of food allergy, such as threats with foods. Bullying has also been associated with decreased quality of life.[56]

In 2013, the federal legislature encouraged states to adopt laws requiring schools to have a supply of "stock" epinephrine autoinjectors available to students who have never had a prior reaction or who have not yet been prescribed an autoinjector by their physician. Five states (California, Nevada, Michigan, Virginia, and North Carolina) have passed laws requiring schools to have "stock" epinephrine available. Most other states have laws or guidelines allowing schools to have "stock" epinephrine but not mandating it. Four states (Pennsylvania, New York, Hawaii, and Iowa) have pending similar legislation. The Centers for Disease Control and Prevention has published *Voluntary Guidelines for Managing Food Allergies in Schools and Early Care and Education Programs* detailing the management of food allergies in these special settings.[57]

Strict avoidance of allergens may not always be advisable as may be the case for some patients with milk and egg allergy. Early studies of baked milk and baked egg tolerance found 75% and 70% to 90% of enrolled children with allergy to milk and egg, respectively, were able to tolerate extensively heated items in an initial oral challenge.[16,58] Subsequently, it has been demonstrated that children who tolerate baked egg and milk seem to become tolerant to the nonbaked forms of these foods more rapidly.[59,60] It is thought that denaturation of conformational protein epitopes from heating causes disrupted epitope recognition by IgE.[61]

FUTURE DIRECTIONS

Clearly, effective therapies for food allergy are desperately needed. Immunotherapy has been proposed as a potentially effective strategy. Clinical trials of various strategies including oral, sublingual, and more recently, epicutaneous routes are encouraging, yet concern for adverse reactions has led to caution and more careful study before widespread implementation.[62] In 1992, a small placebo controlled study of subcutaneous peanut immunotherapy had a relatively high rate of systemic reactions and was subsequently aborted because of a fatality after a placebo subject inadvertently received a maintenance dose of peanut allergen.[63] Preliminary nonrandomized controlled studies indicate that omalizumab may provide a means to reduce adverse reactions and enhance dose escalation in oral immunotherapy with foods.[64–66] Although it appears that immunotherapy may provide protection from accidental exposures, it is unclear whether sustained tolerance is achievable.[67]

Biomarkers that can predict severity of reactions are also urgently needed, so that education and preparedness measures may be focused on those individuals at highest risk. Although component-resolved diagnostics are a step in the right direction, much confusion remains regarding their appropriate use and interpretation, particularly given the geographic differences that have been seen with these tests. The BAT will require more widespread use and evaluation to determine its performance characteristics in predicting severity among widely distributed populations.[38]

SUMMARY

Food-induced anaphylaxis is an important personal and public health concern. Epidemiologic studies have been hampered by the variable presentation of the condition and its diagnosis. Food-induced anaphylaxis seems to affect all ages, but it is most common in children, especially the very young. Although risk factors for severe food-induced reactions are not fully understood, some factors that are associated with fatal outcomes have been uncovered. These factors include having peanut or tree nut allergy, the presence of asthma, especially severe or uncontrolled asthma, lack of access to epinephrine and delay in its administration, failure to assume a supine position during severe reactions, and age, particularly teens and young adults.[10–13] Any food is capable of triggering anaphylaxis. Although peanut, tree nut, and seafood are the most common culprits, cow milk and egg are also capable of inducing severe reactions. Newly recognized allergens that are contained in foods, such as LTP in peaches and α-galin beef, pork, and lamb, seem to be emerging in various geographic areas. Progress is being made in diagnostics for food allergy, such as component-resolved diagnostics and BAT, but more study is needed to understand the role that such tests may have in assessing an individual patient. Although acute treatment of food-induced anaphylaxis is similar to that for other causes, prevention and risk reduction strategies are heavily focused on education, for patients, families, caretakers, and society as a whole.

REFERENCES

1. Clark S, Espinola J, Rudders SA, et al. Frequency of US emergency department visits for food-related acute allergic reactions. J Allergy Clin Immunol 2011;127: 682–3.
2. Clark S, Espinola JA, Rudders SA, et al. Favorable trends in the frequency of U.S. emergency department visits for food allergy, 2001–2009. Allergy Asthma Proc 2013;34:439–45.
3. Liew WK, Williamson E, Tang ML. Anaphylaxis fatalities and admissions in Australia. J Allergy Clin Immunol 2009;123:434–42.
4. Camargo CA Jr, Clark S, Kaplan MS, et al. Regional differences in EpiPen prescriptions in the United States: the potential role of vitamin D. J Allergy Clin Immunol 2007;120:131–6.
5. Mullins RJ, Clark S, Camargo CA Jr. Regional variation in epinephrine autoinjector prescriptions in Australia: more evidence for the vitamin D-anaphylaxis hypothesis. Ann Allergy Asthma Immunol 2009;103:488–95.
6. Sheehan WJ, Graham D, Ma L, et al. Higher incidence of pediatric anaphylaxis in northern areas of the United States. J Allergy Clin Immunol 2009;124:850–2.e2.
7. Rudders SA, Espinola JA, Camargo CA Jr. North-south differences in US emergency department visits for acute allergic reactions. Ann Allergy Asthma Immunol 2010;104:413–6.
8. Jerschow E, Lin RY, Scaperotti MM, et al. Fatal anaphylaxis in the United States, 1999–2010: temporal patterns and demographic associations. J Allergy Clin Immunol 2014;134(6):1318–28.e7.
9. Ford LS, Bloom KA, Nowak-Wegrzyn AH, et al. Basophil reactivity, wheal size, and immunoglobulin levels distinguish degrees of cow's milk tolerance. J Allergy Clin Immunol 2013;131:180–6.e1–3.
10. Bock SA, Munoz-Furlong A, Sampson HA. Fatalities due to anaphylactic reactions to foods. J Allergy Clin Immunol 2001;107:191–3.
11. Pumphrey RS. Fatal posture in anaphylactic shock. J Allergy Clin Immunol 2003; 112:451–2.
12. Bock SA, Munoz-Furlong A, Sampson HA. Further fatalities caused by anaphylactic reactions to food, 2001–2006. J Allergy Clin Immunol 2007;119:1016–8.
13. Pumphrey RS, Gowland MH. Further fatal allergic reactions to food in the United Kingdom, 1999–2006. J Allergy Clin Immunol 2007;119:1018–9.
14. Arena A. Anaphylaxis to apple: is fasting a risk factor for LTP-allergic patients? Eur Ann Allergy Clin Immunol 2010;42:155–8.
15. Cardona V, Luengo O, Garriga T, et al. Co-factor-enhanced food allergy. Allergy 2012;67:1316–8.
16. Nowak-Wegrzyn A, Bloom KA, Sicherer SH, et al. Tolerance to extensively heated milk in children with cow's milk allergy. J Allergy Clin Immunol 2008;122:342–7, 347.e1–2.
17. Asero R, Pravettoni V. Anaphylaxis to plant-foods and pollen allergens in patients with lipid transfer protein syndrome. Curr Opin Allergy Clin Immunol 2013;13: 379–85.
18. Asero R, Antonicelli L, Arena A, et al. Causes of food-induced anaphylaxis in Italian adults: a multi-centre study. Int Arch Allergy Immunol 2009;150:271–7.

19. Romano A, Scala E, Rumi G, et al. Lipid transfer proteins: the most frequent sensitizer in Italian subjects with food-dependent exercise-induced anaphylaxis. Clin Exp Allergy 2012;42:1643–53.
20. Kennedy JL, Stallings AP, Platts-Mills TA, et al. Galactose-alpha-1,3-galactose and delayed anaphylaxis, angioedema, and urticaria in children. Pediatrics 2013;131:e1545–52.
21. Berg EA, Platts-Mills TA, Commins SP. Drug allergens and food–the cetuximab and galactose-alpha-1,3-galactose story. Ann Allergy Asthma Immunol 2014; 112:97–101.
22. Sampson HA, Aceves S, Bock SA, et al. Food allergy: a practice parameter update-2014. J Allergy Clin Immunol 2014;134(5):1016–25.e43.
23. Lee J, Garrett JP, Brown-Whitehorn T, et al. Biphasic reactions in children undergoing oral food challenges. Allergy Asthma Proc 2013;34:220–6.
24. Jarvinen KM, Amalanayagam S, Shreffler WG, et al. Epinephrine treatment is infrequent and biphasic reactions are rare in food-induced reactions during oral food challenges in children. J Allergy Clin Immunol 2009;124:1267–72.
25. Leonard SA, Nowak-Wegrzyn A. Food protein-induced enterocolitis syndrome: an update on natural history and review of management. Ann Allergy Asthma Immunol 2011;107:95–101 [quiz: 62].
26. Bernstein IL, Li JT, Bernstein DI, et al. Allergy diagnostic testing: an updated practice parameter. Ann Allergy Asthma Immunol 2008;100:S1–148.
27. Hamilton RG, Mudd K, White MA, et al. Extension of food allergen specific IgE ranges from the ImmunoCAP to the IMMULITE systems. Ann Allergy Asthma Immunol 2011;107:139–44.
28. Wang J, Godbold JH, Sampson HA. Correlation of serum allergy (IgE) tests performed by different assay systems. J Allergy Clin Immunol 2008;121: 1219–24.
29. Nicolaou N, Poorafshar M, Murray C, et al. Allergy or tolerance in children sensitized to peanut: prevalence and differentiation using component-resolved diagnostics. J Allergy Clin Immunol 2010;125:191–7.e1–13.
30. Klemans RJ, van Os-Medendorp H, Blankestijn M, et al. Diagnostic accuracy of specific IgE to components in diagnosing peanut allergy: a systematic review. Clin Exp Allergy 2014.
31. Lieberman JA, Glaumann S, Batelson S, et al. The utility of peanut components in the diagnosis of IgE-mediated peanut allergy among distinct populations. J Allergy Clin Immunol Pract 2013;1:75–82.
32. Vereda A, van Hage M, Ahlstedt S, et al. Peanut allergy: clinical and immunologic differences among patients from 3 different geographic regions. J Allergy Clin Immunol 2011;127:603–7.
33. Moverare R, Ahlstedt S, Bengtsson U, et al. Evaluation of IgE antibodies to recombinant peanut allergens in patients with reported reactions to peanut. Int Arch Allergy Immunol 2011;156:282–90.
34. Lin YT, Wu CT, Cheng JH, et al. Patterns of sensitization to peanut allergen components in Taiwanese Preschool children. J Microbiol Immunol Infect 2012; 45:90–5.
35. Javaloyes G, Goikoetxea MJ, Garcia Nunez I, et al. Performance of different in vitro techniques in the molecular diagnosis of peanut allergy. J Investig Allergol Clin Immunol 2012;22:508–13.
36. Kattan JD, Sicherer SH, Sampson HA. Clinical reactivity to hazelnut may be better identified by component testing than traditional testing methods. J Allergy Clin Immunol Pract 2014;2:633–44.e1.

37. Santos AF, Douiri A, Becares N, et al. Basophil activation test discriminates between allergy and tolerance in peanut-sensitized children. J Allergy Clin Immunol 2014; 134:645–52.

38. Patil SU, Shreffler WG. BATting above average: basophil activation testing for peanut allergy. J Allergy Clin Immunol 2014;134:653–4.

39. Simons FE, Ardusso LR, Bilo MB, et al. International consensus on (ICON) anaphylaxis. World Allergy Organ J 2014;7:9.

40. Muraro A, Roberts G, Worm M, et al. Anaphylaxis: guidelines from the European Academy of Allergy and Clinical Immunology. Allergy 2014;69:1026–45.

41. Lieberman P, Nicklas RA, Oppenheimer J, et al. The diagnosis and management of anaphylaxis practice parameter: 2010 update. J Allergy Clin Immunol 2010; 126:477–80.e1–42.

42. Wang J, Young MC, Nowak-Wegrzyn A. International survey of knowledge of food-induced anaphylaxis. Pediatr Allergy Immunol 2014;25:644–50.

43. Grabenhenrich L, Hompes S, Gough H, et al. Implementation of anaphylaxis management guidelines: a register-based study. PLoS One 2012;7:e35778.

44. Jarvinen KM, Sicherer SH, Sampson HA, et al. Use of multiple doses of epinephrine in food-induced anaphylaxis in children. J Allergy Clin Immunol 2008;122:133–8.

45. Boyce JA, Assa'ad A, Burks AW, et al. Guidelines for the diagnosis and management of food allergy in the United States: report of the NIAID-sponsored expert panel. J Allergy Clin Immunol 2010;126:S1–58.

46. Kim L, Nevis IF, Tsai G, et al. Children under 15 kg with food allergy may be at risk of having epinephrine auto-injectors administered into bone. Allergy Asthma Clin Immunol 2014;10:40.

47. Fleischer DM, Perry TT, Atkins D, et al. Allergic reactions to foods in preschool-aged children in a prospective observational food allergy study. Pediatrics 2012;130:e25–32.

48. Nguyen-Luu NU, Ben-Shoshan M, Alizadehfar R, et al. Inadvertent exposures in children with peanut allergy. Pediatr Allergy Immunol 2012;23:133–9.

49. Kemp SF, Lockey RF, Wolf BL, et al. A review of 266 cases. Arch Intern Med 1995; 155:1749–54.

50. Pieretti MM, Chung D, Pacenza R, et al. Audit of manufactured products: use of allergen advisory labels and identification of labeling ambiguities. J Allergy Clin Immunol 2009;124:337–41.

51. Remington BC, Baumert JL, Marx DB, et al. Quantitative risk assessment of foods containing peanut advisory labeling. Food Chem Toxicol 2013;62: 179–87.

52. Sicherer SH, Sampson HA. Food allergy: epidemiology, pathogenesis, diagnosis, and treatment. J Allergy Clin Immunol 2014;133:291–307 [quiz: 8].

53. Sicherer SH, Furlong TJ, DeSimone J, et al. The US Peanut and Tree Nut Allergy Registry: characteristics of reactions in schools and day care. J Pediatr 2001; 138:560–5.

54. Nowak-Wegrzyn A, Conover-Walker MK, Wood RA. Food-allergic reactions in schools and preschools. Arch Pediatr Adolesc Med 2001;155:790–5.

55. McIntyre CL, Sheetz AH, Carroll CR, et al. Administration of epinephrine for life-threatening allergic reactions in school settings. Pediatrics 2005;116: 1134–40.

56. Shemesh E, Annunziato RA, Ambrose MA, et al. Child and parental reports of bullying in a consecutive sample of children with food allergy. Pediatrics 2013; 131:e10–7.

57. Centers for Disease Control and Prevention. Voluntary guidelines for managing food allergies in schools and early care and education programs. Washington, DC: US Department of Health and Human Services; 2013.

58. Konstantinou GN, Giavi S, Kalobatsou A, et al. Consumption of heat-treated egg by children allergic or sensitized to egg can affect the natural course of egg allergy: hypothesis-generating observations. J Allergy Clin Immunol 2008;122: 414–5.

59. Kim JS, Nowak-Wegrzyn A, Sicherer SH, et al. Dietary baked milk accelerates the resolution of cow's milk allergy in children. J Allergy Clin Immunol 2011;128: 125–31.e2.

60. Leonard SA, Sampson HA, Sicherer SH, et al. Dietary baked egg accelerates resolution of egg allergy in children. J Allergy Clin Immunol 2012;130:473–80.e1.

61. Martos G, Lopez-Exposito I, Bencharitiwong R, et al. Mechanisms underlying differential food allergy response to heated egg. J Allergy Clin Immunol 2011;127: 990–7.e1–2.

62. Nowak-Wegrzyn A, Sampson HA. Future therapies for food allergies. J Allergy Clin Immunol 2011;127:558–73 [quiz: 74–5].

63. Oppenheimer JJ, Nelson HS, Bock SA, et al. Treatment of peanut allergy with rush immunotherapy. J Allergy Clin Immunol 1992;90:256–62.

64. Nadeau KC, Schneider LC, Hoyte L, et al. Rapid oral desensitization in combination with omalizumab therapy in patients with cow's milk allergy. J Allergy Clin Immunol 2011;127:1622–4.

65. Schneider LC, Rachid R, LeBovidge J, et al. A pilot study of omalizumab to facilitate rapid oral desensitization in high-risk peanut-allergic patients. J Allergy Clin Immunol 2013;132:1368–74.

66. Begin P, Dominguez T, Wilson SP, et al. Phase 1 results of safety and tolerability in a rush oral immunotherapy protocol to multiple foods using Omalizumab. Allergy Asthma Clin Immunol 2014;10:7.

67. Anagnostou K, Clark A. Peanut immunotherapy. Clin Transl Allergy 2014;4:30.

68. Celik-Bilgili S, Mehl A, Verstege A, et al. The predictive value of specific immunoglobulin E levels in serum for the outcome of oral food challenges. Clin Exp Allergy 2005;35:268–73.

69. Garcia-Ara C, Boyano-Martinez T, Diaz-Pena JM, et al. Specific IgE levels in the diagnosis of immediate hypersensitivity to cows' milk protein in the infant. J Allergy Clin Immunol 2001;107:185–90.

70. Sampson HA, Ho DG. Relationship between food-specific IgE concentrations and the risk of positive food challenges in children and adolescents. J Allergy Clin Immunol 1997;100:444–51.

71. Boyano Martinez T, Garcia-Ara C, Diaz-Pena JM, et al. Validity of specific IgE antibodies in children with egg allergy. Clin Exp Allergy 2001;31:1464–9.

72. Maloney JM, Rudengren M, Ahlstedt S, et al. The use of serum-specific IgE measurements for the diagnosis of peanut, tree nut, and seed allergy. J Allergy Clin Immunol 2008;122:145–51.

73. Rance F, Abbal M, Lauwers-Cances V. Improved screening for peanut allergy by the combined use of skin prick tests and specific IgE assays. J Allergy Clin Immunol 2002;109:1027–33.

74. Masthoff LJ, Pasmans SG, van Hoffen E, et al. Diagnostic value of hazelnut allergy tests including rCor a 1 spiking in double-blind challenged children. Allergy 2012;67:521–7.

75. Yang AC, Arruda LK, Santos AB, et al. Measurement of IgE antibodies to shrimp tropomyosin is superior to skin prick testing with commercial extract and

measurement of IgE to shrimp for predicting clinically relevant allergic reactions after shrimp ingestion. J Allergy Clin Immunol 2010;125:872–8.

76. Jirapongsananuruk O, Sripramong C, Pacharn P, et al. Specific allergy to Penaeus monodon (seawater shrimp) or Macrobrachium rosenbergii (freshwater shrimp) in shrimp-allergic children. Clin Exp Allergy 2008;38:1038–47.

77. Permaul P, Stutius LM, Sheehan WJ, et al. Sesame allergy: role of specific IgE and skin-prick testing in predicting food challenge results. Allergy Asthma Proc 2009;30:643–8.

78. Sampson HA. Utility of food-specific IgE concentrations in predicting symptomatic food allergy. J Allergy Clin Immunol 2001;107:891–6.

79. Hill DJ, Heine RG, Hosking CS. The diagnostic value of skin prick testing in children with food allergy. Pediatr Allergy Immunol 2004;15:435–41.

80. Peters RL, Allen KJ, Dharmage SC, et al. Skin prick test responses and allergen-specific IgE levels as predictors of peanut, egg, and sesame allergy in infants. J Allergy Clin Immunol 2013;132:874–80.

81. van Veen WJ, Dikkeschei LD, Roberts G, et al. Predictive value of specific IgE for clinical peanut allergy in children: relationship with eczema, asthma, and setting (primary or secondary care). Clin Transl Allergy 2013;3:34.

82. Clark AT, Ewan PW. Interpretation of tests for nut allergy in one thousand patients, in relation to allergy or tolerance. Clin Exp Allergy 2003;33:1041–5.

Anaphylaxis to the Carbohydrate Side Chain Alpha-gal

Thomas A.E. Platts-Mills, MD, PhD, FRS*,
Alexander J. Schuyler, BS, BA, Anubha Tripathi, MD,
Scott P. Commins, MD, PhD

KEYWORDS

- Delayed anaphylaxis • Alpha-gal • Ticks • Red-meat allergy • Cetuximab

KEY POINTS

- In 2007, the monoclonal antibody cetuximab was causing severe hypersensitivity reactions during the first infusion in a region of the southeastern United States.
- Investigation of pretreatment sera established that they contained immunoglobulin (Ig) E against the oligosaccharide galactose-alpha-1,3-galactose (alpha-gal), which is present on the Fab of cetuximab.
- Alpha-gal is a blood group substance of nonprimate mammals.
- These IgE antibodies are also associated with delayed anaphylaxis to red meat (ie, to meat or organs of those animals that carry this oligosaccharide).
- There is now extensive evidence that the primary cause of these IgE antibodies is bites from the tick *Amblyomma americanum* or its larvae.

INTRODUCTION AND HISTORY

When Karl Landsteiner[1] first defined the ABO system, he also recognized a B-like substance on mammalian cells. At that time he reported that all immunocompetent individuals had agglutinating antibodies against this substance. Adsorption of these antibodies against rabbit red cells was part of the proof that rabbit cells can activate the alternate pathway of human complement.[2] This B-like substance is now known to be galactose-alpha-1,3-galactose (alpha-gal), which is structurally similar to the B blood group (**Fig. 1**).[3,4] This carbohydrate is a well-recognized immunologic barrier

Disclosure: The authors have nothing to disclose.
Asthma and Allergic Diseases Center, University of Virginia Health System, Charlottesville, VA, USA
* Corresponding author. Allergy Division, University of Virginia Health System, PO Box 801355, Charlottesville, VA 22908-1355.
E-mail address: tap2z@virginia.edu

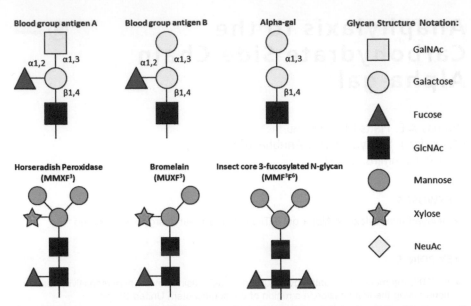

Fig. 1. Glycan structure of blood group antigens and alpha-gal contrasted with those of plant- or insect-related Cross reactive carbohydrate determinants. (*Adapted from* Commins SP, Platts-Mills TA. Anaphylaxis syndromes related to a new mammalian cross-reactive carbohydrate determinant. J Allergy Clin Immunol 2009;124(4):652–57.)

in xenotransplantation. Xenoreactive natural antibodies directed against the alpha-gal moieties on nonprimate mammalian tissue are often implicated in acute organ rejection. One way to circumvent this obstacle may be to raise transgenic organs in pig knockouts lacking the gene expressing alpha-(1,3)-galactosyl transferase, an enzyme inactivated in all primates.[5] It has also been suggested that the antibody response to alpha-gal is as much as 1% of the total immunoglobulin; however, more recent assays in our group suggest a low quantity of immunoglobulin (Ig) G antibodies.[6,7]

The story of IgE to alpha-gal starts in 2006 with 2 anaphylactic reactions to cetuximab in Bentonville, Arkansas, 1 of which was fatal. At the same time, there were 4 observations that were interesting but unexplained:

1. The monoclonal antibody (mAb) cetuximab was causing severe anaphylactic or urticarial reactions in up to 15% of patients treated in Tennessee and North Carolina but not in New York or Boston[8]
2. A patient aged 43 years reported 4 episodes of anaphylaxis, each of which started 4 hours after eating a hamburger (**Box 1**)
3. Sixty percent of the school children in a Kenyan village had serum IgE specific for cat extract, although there were no cats in the village and no relevant allergic symptoms[9]
4. The increasing deer population in rural and suburban Virginia had reached epidemic numbers

At that point, there was no reason to connect these observations and none of them made sense. Investigation of the specificity of the IgE present in the sera of patients before their first cetuximab treatment necessitated the development of an assay for IgE to cetuximab. This assay was simplified because a technique in which the target antigen was biotinylated and then bound to streptavidin ImmunoCAP (Phadia, Portage, MI) had been established in the previous year.[10] At that point, we were

---

Box 1
Delayed, or late night, anaphylaxis to red meat: the presentation and the clinical problem

1. For several years before 2008, patients were presenting to general medicine or allergy clinics for investigation of anaphylaxis or recurrent episodes of urticaria in which the cause was not obvious

2. The histories were striking for onset as an adult, presentation late at night, and/or no apparent acute cause (ie, no bites or stings, no medicines, and no foods within 3 hours of the episode)

3. Most cases had no history of conventional symptoms of food allergy; however, a significant proportion of the cases had made an association with eating beef, pork, or lamb earlier in the day

4. When the patients were tested using a prick test with commercial food extract, including beef, pork, or lamb, they had negative or very small responses (ie, wheals measuring 2–3 mm) to the meats

5. Because of the adult onset, long interval after eating, and negative prick skin tests, many or most of the patients were told they did not have food allergy; nonetheless, they had specific IgE for alpha-gal as well as beef, pork, and lamb

---

approached by Bristol Myers Squibb (BMS) to become involved with the investigation of the reactions to cetuximab.

INVESTIGATION OF THE REACTIONS TO CETUXIMAB: ESTABLISHING THAT THE ANTIGEN ON THAT MOLECULE IS GALACTOSE-ALPHA-1,3-GALACTOSE

The involvement with BMS brought with it connections to ImClone, who manufacture cetuximab, as well as to Dr Chung and the oncology group at Vanderbilt who had pre-treatment sera from patients who had been treated with cetuximab. Many of the sera from Tennessee had IgE antibodies to cetuximab; however, an equal percentage of sera of controls from Tennessee had IgE specific for cetuximab. Thus, it was clear that the presence of these antibodies had everything to do with rural Tennessee and nothing to do with cancer. As an additional control, sera were assayed from a cohort of mothers in Boston (n = 341). In that group, only 1 serum had detectable IgE to cetuximab. Thus, in keeping with the known geographic distribution of reactions to cetuximab, there was good evidence that these antibodies were common in some southern states but rare in northern cities. Among the treated patients, the presence of IgE antibodies to cetuximab of greater than or equal to 0.35 IU/mL was strongly associated with severe reactions during the first infusion (odds ratio, 35).[11]

The next problem was to identify the specificity of the antibodies to this mAb, remembering that they were preexisting. Initially, a wide variety of known allergens including weeds, fungi, and also parasites were considered. Given that other mAbs did not give positive results with these sera it seemed possible that the epitope for these antibodies could be a posttranslational modification of the molecule related to the mouse cell line SP2.0 in which it is expressed. The solution of specificity became easier, because of 2 contributions from ImClone. They provided the same amino acid sequence as cetuximab expressed in Chinese hamster ovary (CHO) cells, a cell line that is not used for the commercial production of cetuximab and is known to produce different glycosylation. In addition, they published the details of the glycosylation of the commercially available cetuximab, which is expressed in a mouse cell line SP2.0.[12] These studies established that the sera with IgE antibodies to cetuximab did not bind to the same antibody expressed in CHO cells, and that the binding was specific for the Fab portion of the molecule. It was Dr Beloo Mirakhur at BMS who first suggested that the target had to be alpha-gal. Full evidence for the specificity was obtained both from direct binding studies and inhibition studies.[11] The target of these IgE antibodies has now been confirmed from studies in Stockholm, Germany, and the Netherlands.[13–15] There is now no doubt that most of the severe reactions to cetuximab are a direct consequence of the presence of IgE to alpha-gal before the first infusion.[11,16]

FURTHER DEVELOPMENTS RELATED TO CETUXIMAB AND OTHER MONOCLONAL ANTIBODIES

In our initial publication, there was a simplistic image of the structure of cetuximab showing the glycosylation sites.[11] Over the next 2 years it became clear that this was not completely accurate. First, the sugars are complex, including diantennary and triantennary complex oligosaccharides with different expressions of alpha-gal (**Fig. 2**).[17] Second, there can be alpha-gal on the Fc portion of the molecule, and, third, in the normal structure of the Fc portion of IgG the glycosylation at Asn299 does not face outwards (see **Fig. 2**).[17,18] Dr Paul Parren and his group at Genmab in Utrecht used sera from Virginia to investigate the presence of relevant sugars on the Fc portion of cetuximab and infliximab. Those results confirmed our main finding that the alpha-gal, which could be identified on the whole molecule, was on the Fab portion of the heavy chain at Asn88. However, when the 2 chains of the Fc were separated using proteinase K there was detectable alpha-gal on the heavy chain.[15]

The combination of these results with other findings made it clear that the glycosylation site on the Fab at Asn88 is a problem, although this glycosylation is not thought to have a significant role in the activity of the molecule. Consequently, the glycosylation site on the Fab at Asn88 has been engineered out of the structure of most new mAbs. Thus, this specific problem is unlikely to arise again. The glycosylation on the Fc portion of IgG molecules plays an important role in defining the binding of IgG to different Fc receptors. It is now possible to engineer the expression of oligosaccharides on these antibodies so that the structure allows binding to different Fc receptors.[18]

DELAYED ANAPHYLAXIS TO RED MEAT

Once the assay for IgE to alpha-gal was established, sera from several different kinds of patients were screened. This screening included patients with histories of asthma, chronic urticaria, atopic dermatitis, and anaphylaxis. The most common history that correlated with IgE to alpha-gal was of urticarial or anaphylactic reactions occurring a few hours after eating red meat, beef, pork, or lamb (see **Box 1**), including the original case and also 2 members of our group. In 2009, we reported 24 cases, all of which had a typical history of delayed urticaria or anaphylaxis and had IgE specific for alpha-gal.[19] In that same year, it was confirmed that the oligosaccharide that Dr Van Hage and her colleagues[20,21] in Sweden had previously identified as an IgE binding epitope on cat IgA was also alpha-gal.

By 2011, about 400 cases of delayed urticaria or anaphylaxis to red meat were known and we evaluated symptoms, lung function, exhaled NO, and serum IgE on ~200 patients. The resulting evidence showed that IgE to alpha-gal had no association with asthma.[22] Thus even patients with high-titer IgE to alpha-gal living in a house with a cat had no increase in their risk of asthma. This finding was surprising because cats, like all mammals, have alpha-gal on many of their proteins and lipids. In contrast, using an assay for alpha-gal, we were not able to detect this antigen airborne in homes with a cat even in the presence of high Fel d 1 levels.[22,23] The studies at that time also examined sera from the Kenyan village and established that the IgE to cat that had been observed earlier was explained by IgE to alpha-gal.[9,22] A recent report on patients in Zimbabwe found that IgE antibodies to alpha-gal were common among patients being evaluated in an allergy clinic.[24] In contrast, the results from Africa have not so far identified cases of meat allergy.

Anaphylactic or urticarial reactions to red meat are well recognized in Australia,[25] which came to light from the original observations of Dr Sherril Van Nunen. In 2006, she had reported to the New South Wales Allergy Society that individuals who had experienced tick bites in the bush were at risk of serious reactions following ingestion of red meat. She published her results in 2009 and related those results to the published evidence about IgE to alpha-gal.[11,19,25] Subsequently, with Dr Mullins we confirmed that the patients with delayed reactions to red meat in Australia had IgE antibodies specific for alpha-gal.[26] Cases of reactions to red meat have now been identified in France, Sweden, Germany, Japan, and Australia as well as in the United States (**Fig. 3**A, **Table 1**).[27–34]

THE EVIDENCE THAT TICKS PLAY AN IMPORTANT ROLE AND ARE POSSIBLY THE ONLY SIGNIFICANT CAUSE OF IMMUNOGLOBULIN E RESPONSES TO GALACTOSE-ALPHA-1,3-GALACTOSE IN THE UNITED STATES

The speed with which new cases of delayed anaphylaxis to red meat (DARM) have been diagnosed in the United States strongly suggests that the condition has increased over the last 10 years. Although it is difficult to prove that a disease that was not previously recognized has increased, the reintroduction of deer to the east coast and the subsequent dramatic increase in the deer population provides a possible explanation for the increase in cases. The white-tailed, or Virginia, deer (*Odocoileus virginianus*), which nearly became extinct in large areas of the east coast in 1930, is a major host for ticks. These deer were reintroduced to the Blue Ridge Mountains around 1950, and their numbers have been increasing rapidly since then. Thus it is plausible that the dramatic increase in the deer population, particularly close to residential areas, has played a major role in increasing exposure to the lone star tick and its larvae.[35]

The initial reason for suspecting tick bites in the United States was that the areas of the 2 diseases associated with IgE to alpha-gal seemed to be similar to the area with maximum incidence of Rocky Mountain spotted fever.[36–38] That disease is transmitted by 2 species of ticks: *Dermacentor variabilis* (the brown dog tick) and *Amblyomma americanum* (the lone star tick) (see **Fig. 3**B, **Table 2**). The lone star tick has been spreading rapidly in the United States and is being followed by the US Centers for Disease Control and Prevention because it is the major vector for ehrlichiosis.[36,37]

The evidence for tick bites as a major cause of IgE to alpha-gal comes from several observations (**Box 2**). First, we have documented increases in IgE antibodies after tick bites in 4 subjects. Second, there is a significant correlation between reports of prolonged itching after tick bites and the presence of IgE antibodies to alpha-gal in the serum. Bites of larval lone star ticks, like adult ticks, can be intensely pruritic. Bites from the deer tick *Ixodes scapularis*, which transmits Lyme disease, do not generally induce a pruritic skin response; itching after tick bites has been associated with a decrease in the risk of developing positive Lyme serology.[39] Third, there is an excellent correlation between IgE to alpha-gal and IgE to extract of the lone star tick ($r = 0.75$; $P<.001$).[38] In addition, evidence from the group in Stockholm showing the presence of alpha-gal in the gut of the tick and a similar correlation with tick bites in southern

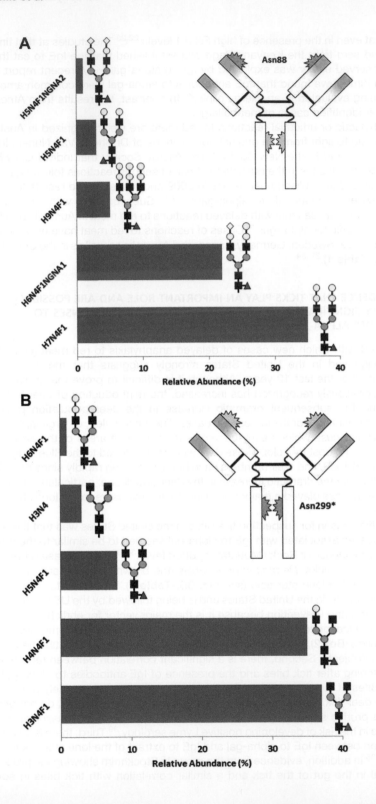

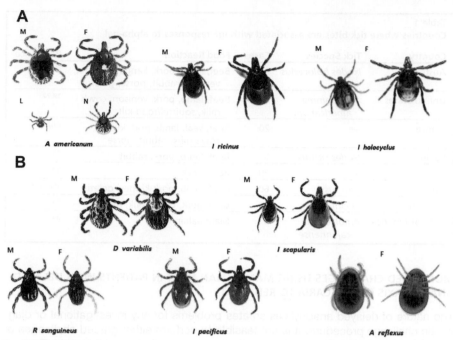

Fig. 3. (*A*) Tick species in which bites are associated with IgE response to alpha-gal. (*B*) Tick species associated with common tick-borne diseases or tick bite anaphylaxis. *A reflexus*, *Argas reflexus*; F, female; L, larva; M, male; N, nymph; *R*, *Rhipicephalus*. (Images of A americanum, D variabilis, I scapularius, R sanguineus, and I pacificus courtesy of University of Rhode Island TickEncounter Resource Center, http://www.tickencounter.org/; with permission.)

Sweden[33] has strengthened this correlation. In addition, subjects living in areas void of ticks do not have IgE to alpha-gal.[11,22,33] The lone star tick is the only tick in the United States whose larvae bite humans, and in several cases we have found high-titer IgE antibodies to alpha-gal following bites from larval ticks. These larval ticks are often known as seed ticks or chiggers. Given the evidence of bites of the lone star tick giving rise to this IgE response, the question becomes why does this tick give rise to such dramatic IgE responses and why are they directed at this oligosaccharide? The problem is in understanding whether this response has more in common with other responses to oligosaccharides (which are usually IgM) or with IgE responses to proteins. There is increasing evidence that the skin can be an important route for IgE antibody responses to proteins such as peanut and wheat.[40,41] However, with those antigens neither the route through which it enters the skin nor the time frame from exposure to antibody response is known.

Fig. 2. Relative abundance of glycosylation patterns on cetuximab at sites Asn88 (*A*) and Asn299 (*B*) as resolved by mass spectroscopy. The blue sections on the Fab arms indicate the murine segments of the antibody. (*Asterisk*) Alpha-gal is not exposed in the intact molecule. See **Fig. 1** for glycan structure notation. (*Adapted from* Ayoub D, Jabs W, Resemann A, et al. Correct primary structure assessment and extensive glyco-profiling of cetuximab by a combination of intact, middle-up, middle-down and bottom-up ESI and MALDI mass spectrometry techniques. MAbs 2013;5(5):699–710.)

Table 1
Countries where tick bites are associated with IgE responses to alpha-gal

Country	Tick Species	Cases	Food Reaction	Reference
Australia	*Ixodes holocyclus*	+400	Beef, lamb, pork, kangaroo, goat, venison, rabbit, horse, gelatin	25,26
United States	*Amblyomma americanum*	>1000	Beef, lamb, pork, venison, cow's milk, squirrel/road kill	19,22
France	—	20	Beef, veal, lamb, pork kidney, cow's milk, rabbit, horse	27,28
Spain	*Ixodes ricinus*	5	Beef, lamb, pork, rabbit	29
Japan	—	29	Beef, pork	30
Germany	*I ricinus*	60	Beef, lamb, pork kidney, gelatin	14,31,32
Sweden	*I ricinus*	40	Beef, pork, cow's milk, moose	33
Central America	*Amblyomma cajennense*	4	Mammalian meat	34

MONITORED CHALLENGES USING MAMMALIAN MEAT IN PATIENTS WITH DELAYED ANAPHYLAXIS OR URTICARIA TO RED MEAT

The nature of delayed anaphylaxis creates problems for any investigational or diagnostic challenge procedure. It is not feasible to perform either graded challenges or placebo-controlled challenges to investigate reactions that can take up to 6 hours. Our protocol involves a single dose of meat product and most of these studies were performed on patients who reported delayed episodes of urticaria. The potential risk of more severe reactions (eg, anaphylaxis) presents an additional layer of difficulty to diagnostic challenges because most patients are male in an age range in which creating a risk of anaphylaxis or the need for epinephrine is not appropriate. Accordingly, the studies were not performed on patients who reported previous episodes of anaphylaxis and were restricted to subjects less than 50 years of age in order to reduce the risk of the reactions or the use of epinephrine.[32,42]

Table 2
Causal organisms and tick species involved with the transmission of common tick-borne diseases or the less common tick bite anaphylaxis

Tick-borne Disease	Causal Organism	Implicated Tick
Lyme disease	*Borrelia burgdorferi* (United States) *Borrelia afzelii* and *Borrelia garinii* (Europe)	*Ixodes scapularis* and other *Ixodes* spp
Rocky Mountain spotted fever	*Rickettsia rickettsii*	*D variabilis, Rhipicephalus sanguineus, A americanum*
Human monocytic ehrlichiosis	*Ehrlichia chaffeensis*	*A americanum*
Human granulocytic anaplasmosis	*Anaplasma phagocytophilum*	*Ixodes* spp
Anaphylaxis caused by tick bites	Tick saliva	*Argas reflexus* (Europe) *Ixodes holocyclus* (Australia) *R sanguineus* (Brazil) *Ixodes pacificus* (United States)

Box 2
Evidence that tick bites are a cause, or the major cause, of IgE responses to alpha-gal

1. The area of the United States where the IgE antibodies are common coincides with the distribution of the lone star tick
2. A large proportion of patients with these antibodies report prolonged itching after tick bites
3. In 4 cases we have followed increases in IgE antibodies to alpha-gal after tick bites
4. IgE to alpha-gal correlates strongly with IgE to extract of the lone star tick
5. In other countries, bites of ticks of other species have been associated with IgE to alpha-gal
6. Among populations living in large cities of the United States or the extreme north of Sweden where ticks are not present, IgE antibodies to alpha-gal are absent

IgE antibodies to alpha-gal can be measured with cetuximab on a streptavidin Immuno CAP (see Ref.[10]). The assay is also available commercially from IBT/Viracor (Lee's Summit, MO).

Monitored challenges have now been reported from France, Germany, and the United States.[28,32,42] Our challenge results involved 12 cases and 13 controls **(Table 3)**. In 10 cases, there was a significant clinical response involving the skin and, in 1 of these cases, severe intestinal spasms as well. Three of the cases had an increase of serum tryptase level at the time of the skin reaction (ie, 2.5 to 5 hours after eating meat). All the patients who developed urticaria received antihistamines and in 2 cases the symptoms required epinephrine.[42] None of the controls had any symptoms and none of them received any treatment.

To investigate the mechanism of the delayed reaction, we also monitored patients' basophil levels during the challenge to investigate the activation of these cells as judged by upregulation of CD63. For the basophil studies the cells were fixed ex vivo without further stimulation. Ten of the alpha-gal IgE-positive subjects had significant upregulation of CD63 starting at 3 hours or later, which broadly correlated with the timing of the skin reactions. Surprisingly, 5 of the 13 controls showed significant upregulation of CD63 ex vivo at the same time (ie, 3–5 hours after eating meat).[42] We assumed that this upregulation reflects the time at which significant alpha-gal

Table 3
Red meat challenges in patients with or without IgE specific for alpha-gal

Group	Time to Symptoms (h)	Urticaria[a]	Antihistamine	Epinephrine	Prednisone	Tryptase Level Increase
Allergic (n = 12)	2.45–5.00	10 of 12[b]	9 of 12	2 of 12	4 of 12	3 of 11[c]
Controls (n = 13)	NR	0 of 13[d]	0 of 13	0 of 13	0 of 13	0 of 13

Abbreviation: NR, not reported.
[a] Urticaria was characterized by flushing.
[b] Flushing with intestinal spasms was observed in only 1 of these subjects.
[c] Tryptase level increase: (1) 4.7 to 10.7 ng/mL, (2) 4.2 to 20.1 ng/mL, (3) 6.2 to 18.3 ng/mL.
[d] $P<.001$.
Data from Commins SP, James H, Stevens W, et al. Delayed clinical and ex vivo response to mammalian meat in patients with IgE to galactose-alpha-1,3-galactose. J Allergy Clin Immunol 2014;134:108–15.

enters the circulation. However, there is published evidence that basophils have a receptor for very-low-density lipoprotein (VLDL) and low-density lipoprotein (LDL) that can trigger histamine release.[43,44] Our current hypothesis is that the delay in the clinical response is best explained by the time needed for absorption of lipids and glycolipids as chylomicrons and the subsequent processing to VLDL and LDL.

In the Alsace region of France and the north eastern region of Germany, 2 separate groups have described cases of DARM.[27,28,31,32] In both areas they have identified pork kidney as an important cause of the naturally occurring reactions as well as an excellent agent for inducing reactions in the context of diagnostic challenges. In each case, the reactions were more severe and also more rapid with the kidney challenge. However, even with pork kidney none of the patients reported immediate (ie, within 20 minutes) oral symptoms.

A large proportion of patients report that their responses are not only delayed but that they are also inconsistent. Some patients report that responses occur more consistently if they take alcohol at the same time as the meat. Recently, the Biedermann group in Germany also reported that the response to pork kidney can be enhanced with exercise, aspirin, and/or alcohol.[32] The important question at this point is to establish what form of the glycolipid enters the circulation 2 to 5 hours after eating mammalian meat or organs, such as kidney, heart, stomach, or liver from nonprimate mammals.

SUMMARY

Two different and novel forms of anaphylaxis have now been associated with IgE to alpha-gal. Reactions to cetuximab continue to occur, including a fatal reaction that occurred during the first infusion in a 40-year-old patient with colon cancer in August of 2014.[11,16] In addition, severe delayed anaphylactic reactions to red meat continue to occur in patients who were not aware of being allergic, or had been dismissed by a physician because the physician did not think that the reactions could take 4 hours. In 2014, we reported a case of severe anaphylaxis to pork in a previously nonatopic 73-year-old woman.[45]

The characteristic features of the syndrome of DARM are late onset of urticarial or anaphylactic episodes, together with no immediate cause, a history of pruritic tick bites, and exposure to red meat 3 to 5 hours before the onset of symptoms. However, many cases are less obvious, with longer delays, no clear history of tick bites and symptoms such as gastrointestinal spasm alone, or just facial swelling. In some areas of the United States it is normal practice to test otherwise unexplained cases of anaphylaxis. In central Virginia IgE to alpha-gal is now the most common cause of anaphylaxis in adults. Among city dwellers the syndrome is rare, but nonetheless the syndrome needs to be on the list of possible causes of otherwise unexplained anaphylaxis.

The evidence about ticks as a cause of the IgE response is good but does not exclude a role for other parasitic exposures. Ticks in other countries are not the same. In Australia the relevant tick is *Ixodes holocyclus*, whereas in Europe the relevant tick is *Ixodes ricinus* (see **Fig. 3**). The group of investigators in Stockholm has shown that *I ricinus* has alpha-gal in its gastrointestinal tract.[13] In our experience, alpha-gal IgE titers seem to diminish over time with avoidance of ticks, although there is neither a regular time course for this loss of sensitivity nor a guaranteed reduction in symptom severity among all patients. In contrast, continued exposure to ticks seems to augment the already existing IgE antibody response. The important question is how these ticks induce an IgE responses and why it is directed against this specific oligosaccharide.

Table 4
Allergic diseases in which the route of sensitization is not the same as the route of exposure giving symptoms

Allergic Syndrome	Presentation	Route of Sensitization	Mechanism
Oral allergy syndrome	Oral symptoms; eg, to apple, cherries, hazelnut	Sensitization to inhaled pollen; eg, birch	Cross reactivity between Bet v 1 and major allergens; eg, Mal d 1, Pru av 1, Cor a 1
Pork/cat syndrome	Oral symptoms and anaphylaxis to pork	Sensitization to cat albumin (Fel d 2)	Cross reactivity between albumins of cat and pork
Peanut allergy	Anaphylactic reactions to oral peanut	Sensitization through the skin in patients with a filaggrin defect	Sensitization to Ara h 1 and Ara h 2
DARM	Delayed urticarial and anaphylactic reactions to red meat	Sensitization to alpha-gal from tick bites	Sensitization to mammalian oligosaccharide alpha-gal

One of the striking things about the syndrome is that the route of exposure to the antigen is via the skin, whereas the symptoms follow oral exposure. This difference adds to an increasing list of allergic diseases in which the route of initial exposure is not the same as the site of the symptoms (Table 4). In addition, the delay in reaction after eating meat adds to the group of conditions in which oral exposure seems to be causal and IgE antibodies are involved but the patient cannot identify the relevant food or food groups via more immediate, oral symptoms (ie, pruritus or swelling).[41,46,47] None of these conditions can be evaluated using double-blind placebo-controlled challenges.

The evolution in understanding of DARM has important implications in understanding and treating IgE-mediated hypersensitivity. No feature of the disease was obvious to allergists in practice, including to those who now study it. Most adult patients who reported reactions occurring 4 hours or more after eating meat and had negative or very small prick test responses to the relevant meat were informed that this could not be IgE-mediated hypersensitivity to the food. Furthermore, histories that included previous tick bites were thought to be irrelevant. In addition, the role of the increasing deer population in suburban areas of the east coast focuses attention on the many ways in which changes in human behavior have affected allergic disease.

REFERENCES

1. Landsteiner K. Specificity of serological reactions. Baltimore (MD): Charles C Thomas; 1936.
2. Platts-Mills TA, Ishizaka K. Activation of the alternate pathway of human complements by rabbit cells. J Immunol 1974;113(1):348–58.
3. Milland J, Sandrin MS. ABO blood group and related antigens, natural antibodies and transplantation. Tissue Antigens 2006;68:459–66.
4. Macher BA, Galili U. The Galalpha1,3Galbeta1,4GlcNAc-R (alpha-Gal) epitope: a carbohydrate of unique evolutionary and clinical relevance. Biochim Biophys Acta 2008;1780:75–88.

5. Koike C, Uddin M, Wildman DE, et al. Functionally important glycosyltransferase gain and loss during catarrhine primate emergence. Proc Natl Acad Sci U S A 2007;104:559–64.

6. Galili U. The alpha-gal epitope and the anti-Gal antibody in xenotransplantation and in cancer immunotherapy. Immunol Cell Biol 2005;83(6):674–86.

7. Rispens T, Derksen NI, Commins SP, et al. IgE production to alpha-gal is accompanied by elevated levels of specific IgG1 antibodies and low amounts of IgE to blood group B. PLoS One 2013;8(2):e55566.

8. O'Neil BH, Allen R, Spigel DR, et al. High incidence of cetuximab-related infusion reactions in Tennessee and North Carolina and the association with atopic history. J Clin Oncol 2007;25:3644–8.

9. Perzanowski MS, Ng'ang'a LW, Carter MC, et al. Atopy, asthma, and antibodies to *Ascaris* among rural and urban children in Kenya. J Pediatr 2002;140(5):582–8.

10. Erwin EA, Custis NJ, Satinover SM, et al. Quantitative measurement of IgE antibodies to purified allergens using streptavidin linked to a high-capacity solid phase. J Allergy Clin Immunol 2005;115:1029–35.

11. Chung CH, Mirakhur B, Chan E, et al. Cetuximab-induced anaphylaxis and IgE specific for galactose-alpha-1,3-galactose. N Engl J Med 2008;358:1109–17.

12. Qian J, Liu T, Yang L, et al. Structural characterization of N-linked oligosaccharides on monoclonal antibody cetuximab by the combination of orthogonal matrix-assisted laser desorption/ionization hybrid quadrupole-quadrupole time-of-flight tandem mass spectrometry and sequential enzymatic digestion. Anal Biochem 2007;364:8–18.

13. Hamsten C, Starkhammar M, Tran TA, et al. Identification of galactose-alpha-1,3-galactose in the gastrointestinal tract of the tick *Ixodes ricinus*; possible relationship with red meat allergy. Allergy 2013;68(4):549–52.

14. Jappe U. Update on meat allergy. alpha-Gal: a new epitope, a new entity? Hautarzt 2012;63(4):299–306 [in German].

15. Lammerts van Bueren JJ, Rispens T, Verploegen S, et al. Anti-galactose-alpha-1,3-galactose IgE from allergic patients does not bind alpha-galactosylated glycans on intact therapeutic antibody Fc domains. Nat Biotechnol 2011;29(7):574–6.

16. Maier S, Chung C, Morse M, et al. A retrospective analysis of cross-reacting cetuximab IgE antibody and its association with severe infusion reactions. Cancer Med 2014;9(10):333.

17. Ayoub D, Jabs W, Resemann A, et al. Correct primary structure assessment and extensive glyco-profiling of cetuximab by a combination of intact, middle-up, middle-down and bottom-up ESI and MALDI mass spectrometry techniques. MAbs 2013;5(5):699–710.

18. Hayes J, Cosgave E, Struwe W, et al. Glycosylation and Fc receptors. Curr Top Microbiol Immunol 2014;382:165–99.

19. Commins SP, Satinover SM, Hosen J, et al. Delayed anaphylaxis, angioedema, or urticaria after consumption of red meat in patients with IgE antibodies specific for galactose-alpha-1,3-galactose. J Allergy Clin Immunol 2009;123:426–33.

20. Adedoyin J, Gronlund H, Oman H, et al. Cat IgA, representative of new carbohydrate cross-reactive allergens. J Allergy Clin Immunol 2007;119(3):640–5.

21. Gronlund H, Adedoyin J, Commins SP, et al. The carbohydrate galactose-alpha-1,3-galactose is a major IgE-binding epitope on cat IgA. J Allergy Clin Immunol 2009;123(5):1189–91.

22. Commins SP, Kelly LA, Ronmark E, et al. Galactose-alpha-1,3-galactose-specific IgE is associated with anaphylaxis but not asthma. Am J Respir Crit Care Med 2012;185:723–30.

23. Platts-Mills JA, Custis NJ, Woodfolk JA, et al. Airborne endotoxin in homes with domestic animals: implications for cat-specific tolerance. J Allergy Clin Immunol 2005;116(2):384–9.
24. Arkestal K, Sibanda E, Thors C, et al. Impaired allergy diagnostics among parasite-infected patients caused by IgE antibodies to the carbohydrate epitope galactose-alpha 1,3-galactose. J Allergy Clin Immunol 2011;127(4):1024–8.
25. Van Nunen SA, O'Connor KS, Clarke LR, et al. An association between tick bite reactions and red meat allergy in humans. Med J Aust 2009;190:510–1.
26. Mullins RJ, James H, Platts-Mills TA, et al. Relationship between red meat allergy and sensitization to gelatin and galactose-alpha-1,3-galactose. J Allergy Clin Immunol 2012;129:1334–42.e1.
27. Jacquenet S, Moneret-Vautrin DA, Bihain BE. Mammalian meat-induced anaphylaxis: clinical relevance of anti-galactose-alpha-1,3-galactose IgE confirmed by means of skin tests to cetuximab. J Allergy Clin Immunol 2009; 124(3):603–5.
28. Morisset M, Richard C, Astier C, et al. Anaphylaxis to pork kidney is related to IgE antibodies specific for galactose-alpha-1,3-galactose. Allergy 2012;67: 699–704.
29. Nunez R, Carballada F, Gonzalez-Quintela A, et al. Delayed mammalian meat-induced anaphylaxis due to galactose-alpha-1,3-galactose in 5 European patients. J Allergy Clin Immunol 2011;128(5):1122–4.e1.
30. Takahashi H, Chinuki Y, Tanaka A, et al. Laminin y-1 and collagen x-1 (VI) chain are galactose-a-1,3-galactose-bound allergens in beef. Allergy 2014;69:199–207.
31. Caponetto P, Fischer J, Biedermann T. Gelatin-containing sweets can elicit anaphylaxis in a patient with sensitization to galactose-α-1,3-galactose. J Allergy Clin Immunol Pract 2013;1(3):302–3.
32. Fischer J, Hebsaker J, Caponetto P, et al. Galactose-alpha-1,3-galactose sensitization is a prerequisite for pork-kidney allergy and cofactor-related mammalian meat anaphylaxis. J Allergy Clin Immunol 2014;133(3):755–9.e1.
33. Hamsten C, Tran T, Starkhammar M, et al. Red meat allergy in Sweden: association with tick sensitization and B-negative blood groups. J Allergy Clin Immunol 2013;132(6):1431–4.
34. Wickner P, Commins S. The first 4 Central American cases of delayed meat allergy with galactose-alpha-1,3-galactose positivity clustered among field biologists in Panama. J Allergy Clin Immunol 2014;133(2);Supplement, AB212.
35. Pound J, Lohmeyer K, Davey R, et al. Efficacy of amitraz-impregnated collars on white-tailed deer (Artiodactyla: Cervidae) in reducing free-living populations of lone star ticks (Acari: Ixodidae). J Econ Entomol 2012;105(6):2207–12.
36. Stein K, Waterman M, Waldon J. The effects of vegetation density and habitat disturbance on the spatial distribution of ixodid ticks (Acari: Ixodidae). Geospat Health 2008;2(2):241–52.
37. Romero C. Reportable disease surveillance in Virginia, 2012. Richmond (VA): Virginia Department of Health; 2012.
38. Commins S, James H, Kelly E, et al. The relevance of tick bites to the production of IgE antibodies to the mammalian oligosaccharide galactose-α-1,3-galactose. J Allergy Clin Immunol 2011;127:1286–93.
39. Burke G, Wikel SK, Spielman A, et al, Tick-borne Infection Study Group. Hypersensitivity to ticks and Lyme disease risk. Emerg Infect Dis 2005;11:36–41.
40. Brough H, Simpson A, Makinson K, et al. Peanut allergy: effect on environmental peanut exposure in children with filaggrin loss-of-function mutations. J Allergy Clin Immunol 2014;134(4):867–75.

41. Yokooji T, Kurihara S, Murakami T, et al. Characterization of causative allergens for wheat-dependent exercise-induced anaphylaxis sensitized with hydrolyzed wheat proteins in facial soap. Allergol Int 2013;64(4):435–45.
42. Commins SP, James H, Stevens W, et al. Delayed clinical and ex vivo response to mammalian meat in patients with IgE to galactose-alpha-1,3-galactose. J Allergy Clin Immunol 2014;134:108–15.
43. Gonen B, O'Donnell P, Post T, et al. Very low density lipoproteins (VLDL) trigger the release of histamine from human basophils. Biochim Biophys Acta 1987; 917(3):418–24.
44. Virgolini I, Li S, Yang Q, et al. Characterization of LDL and VLDL binding sites on human basophils and mast cells. Arterioscler Thromb Vasc Biol 1995;15(1): 17–26.
45. Tripathi A, Commins SP, Heymann P, et al. Delayed anaphylaxis to red meat masquerading as idiopathic anaphylaxis. J Allergy Clin Immunol Pract 2014; 2(3):259–65.
46. Erwin EA, James HR, Gutekunst HM, et al. Serum IgE measurement and detection of food allergy in pediatric patients with eosinophilic esophagitis. Ann Allergy Asthma Immunol 2010;104(6):496–502.
47. Brockow K, Kneissl D, Valentini L, et al. Using a gluten oral food challenge protocol to improve diagnosis of wheat-dependent exercise-induced anaphylaxis. J Allergy Clin Immunol 2014.

Exercise-Induced Anaphylaxis

Anna M. Feldweg, MD

KEYWORDS

- Exercise-induced anaphylaxis • Food-dependent exercise-induced anaphylaxis
- Omega-5-gliadin • Cromolyn sodium • Cholinergic urticaria

KEY POINTS

- Symptoms of exercise-induced anaphylaxis/food-dependent exercise-induced anaphylaxis include extreme fatigue, warmth, flushing, pruritus, and urticaria, progressing to angioedema, wheezing, upper airway obstruction, and collapse.
- Diagnosis of exercise-induced anaphylaxis/food-dependent exercise-induced anaphylaxis is usually based on the clinical history and exclusion of other disorders.
- Exercise challenge (with or without food) is useful when positive, but the symptoms can be difficult to elicit, and the diagnosis can be made without this maneuver. In food-dependent exercise-induced anaphylaxis, allergen-specific immunoglobulin E to the culprit food should be demonstrable.
- Management includes education about safe conditions for exercise, the importance of ceasing exercise immediately if symptoms develop, appropriate use of epinephrine and, for patients with food-dependent exercise-induced anaphylaxis, avoidance of the culprit food for at least 4 hours before exercise.
- All patients should be equipped with epinephrine for self-administration. H1 antihistamines may reduce symptoms in some patients but do not prevent attacks. Oral cromolyn sodium seems to be useful in many cases of food-dependent exercise-induced anaphylaxis. Refractory cases have been treated with misoprostol or omalizumab.

INTRODUCTION

Exercise-induced anaphylaxis (ElAn) is a disorder in which anaphylaxis occurs exclusively in association with physical exertion. Food-dependent exercise-induced anaphylaxis (FDEIAn) is a similar disorder in which symptoms develop only if exertion takes place within a few hours of eating, and usually only if a certain food(s) is ingested, to which the patient is sensitized.

The author has nothing to disclose.
Division of Rheumatology, Immunology, and Allergy, Brigham and Women's Hospital, Harvard Medical School, 1 Jimmy Fund Way, Smith Building, 6th Floor, Boston, MA 02115, USA
E-mail address: AFELDWEG@PARTNERS.ORG

Immunol Allergy Clin N Am 35 (2015) 261–275
http://dx.doi.org/10.1016/j.iac.2015.01.005   immunology.theclinics.com
0889-8561/15/$ – see front matter © 2015 Elsevier Inc. All rights reserved.

EPIDEMIOLOGY

ElAn and FDElAn have been reported around the world and in patients of all ages, although adolescents and young adults make up most cases in the literature.[1-5] Both ElAn and FDElAn seem to be rare. In one of the few studies of prevalence, rates of 0.03% and 0.017%, for ElAn and FDElAn, respectively, were estimated among Japanese adolescents.[3] However, in the author's clinical experience, FDElAn is more common than ElAn. Slightly more females than males have been reported to be affected.[6] Most cases of ElAn and FDElAn are sporadic, although there are rare reports of familial cases.[7,8]

SYMPTOMS AND CLINICAL FEATURES

In both ElAn and FDElAN, episodes of symptoms are unpredictable in most patients in that a given level of physical exertion may trigger symptoms on one occasion but not on other similar occasions. Most patients exercise routinely but only develop attacks occasionally.

The signs and symptoms are similar to those in anaphylaxis from other causes. A typical episode begins while the patient is exercising vigorously, with a sensation of warmth and flushing, sometimes accompanied by sudden fatigue.[9,10] The individual then becomes aware of pruritus, and urticaria often begins to appear on the skin. If the episode progresses (because the patient continues the exercise), lightheadedness or presyncope, gastrointestinal symptoms (nausea, abdominal cramps, diarrhea), angioedema (typically of the face or hands), throat tightness, or bronchospastic symptoms may develop. In severe episodes, patients become hypotensive and collapse. After an episode of ElAn or FDElAn, patients may report fatigue or headache lasting a day or so.[10,11]

If the patient stops the activity immediately at the first awareness of symptoms, there is most often improvement or resolution of the symptoms within minutes. However, not all patients instinctively stop what they are doing. Some may try to "push through" to see if the symptoms will pass, and others may become frightened and try to reach a place where there are other people. Runners may sprint for home. "Pushing through" uniformly results in a worsening of symptoms, and discussing this with patients is an important part of initial management.

Triggering Forms of Exercise

Vigorous forms of exercise, such as jogging, sports involving sudden bursts of sprinting (soccer/football), dancing, and aerobics are most likely to trigger symptoms.[11] However, brisk walking or yard work can trigger episodes in some patients, and there are case reports of older adults in whom the physical exertion of crossing a road was sufficient.[12]

Food-dependent Exercise-induced Anaphylaxis

In FDElAn, symptoms occur only when the person exercises within minutes to a few hours after eating. In rare cases, symptoms occur when the food is eaten in the minutes immediately after exercise.[13] Patients describe episodes in which the combination of the food and exercise precipitates attacks: they can eat the food in question without symptoms if there is no associated exercise, and they can exercise without symptoms if they have not eaten the culprit food. Most patients have symptoms only after eating a specific food, although a few have attacks if any food (usually solids rather than liquids) has been ingested.[14] Rare patients have been described in whom symptoms only occurred if 2 foods were eaten together before exercise,[15] or who only react to the food in a certain form (eg, tofu vs soy milk).[16] The amount of food ingested may be important in some patients.[17,18]

The foods most commonly implicated in FDEIAn are wheat, other grains, and nuts in Western populations and wheat and shellfish in Asian populations; however, an array of culprit foods has been reported, including fruits, vegetables, seeds, legumes, and, less often, various meats, cow's milk, and egg.[1,19–21] Patients should have IgE specific to the culprit food, although this is sometimes difficult to show with standard skin testing or in vitro IgE immunoassays (see later discussion).

Other Factors That May Facilitate Symptoms

Many patients have symptoms more readily in the presence of one or more additional co-triggers, although exercise remains the immediate inciting factor. These include the following:

- Nonsteroidal antiinflammatory drugs (NSAIDs)[18,22–25]
- Alcoholic beverages[11,18]
- Premenstrual or ovulatory phases of the menstrual cycle in women[26,27]
- Extremes of temperature (either high heat and humidity or cold exposure)[11]
- Seasonal pollen exposure in pollen-sensitized patients[11]

THEORIES OF PATHOGENESIS

As in other forms of anaphylaxis, mast cell activation and release of various mediators are believed to be responsible for the signs and symptoms of EIAn and FDEIAn, based on skin biopsies showing mast cell degranulation[28] and demonstration of transient elevations in plasma histamine[29,30] and serum tryptase after episodes.[31,32] However, the specific changes that occur during exercise and that lead to symptoms, in the presence of food or independent of it, remain unclear. The role of basophils has not been studied. Theories of pathogenesis are summarized in **Table 1**.

Recent work by investigators in Germany and Japan has shed new light on the pathogenesis of FDEIAn and suggest that this disorder represents a primary food allergy, in which symptoms develop only in the presence of various co-triggers, of which exercise is one but not necessarily an essential one.[18] In a study of 16 patients with wheat-dependent FDEIAn and sensitization to omega-5 gliadin (an allergenic protein in gluten and the best-characterized allergen in wheat-dependent FDEIAn), subjects underwent successive challenges with increasing amounts of gluten-rich bread, combined with alcohol, aspirin, and finally exercise if symptoms did not develop with the other factors. Alcohol, aspirin, and exercise are all known to increase gastric or intestinal permeability. In 14 of 16 subjects, symptoms developed with some combination of the bread, alcohol, and aspirin, without exercise, suggesting that exercise is simply another co-trigger that can augment the clinical expression of an underlying food allergy, rather than an absolute requirement for symptoms. The investigators suggested that the term *augmentation factor–triggered food allergy* might be more accurate than FDEIAn.

DIAGNOSIS

The diagnosis of EIAn or FDEIAn can usually be made clinically, based on a meticulous history of the events surrounding each episode and exclusion of other disorders that could present similarly (**Table 2**).

Important components of the clinical history, physical examination, and laboratory testing, and issues surrounding exercise testing are summarized below.

Table 1
Theories of pathogenesis for EIAn and FDEIAn

Disorder	Proposed Mechanism	References
EIAn	Abnormalities related to mast cell secretagogues released during exercise (gastrin, endogenous endorphins)	33–35
FDEIAn	Increased gastric/intestinal permeability during exercise leads to abnormal entry of allergens into the circulation only during exercise. Concomitant intake of NSAIDs, which increase gastric permeability, increases the likelihood of symptoms in patients with FDEIAn and supports this mechanism	18,23,36,37
	Exercise mobilizes or activates immune cells from gut-associated depots, stimulating proinflammatory responses that are normally countered by antiinflammatory responses when patient is at rest	38
	Exercise results in alterations in blood flow, redirecting blood from away from the viscera to the skin and musculature. This could carry food allergens to tissues containing mast cells that are not tolerant to those allergens, resulting in an allergic reaction during exercise but not at rest.	39
	Patients with FDEIAn may have dysregulation of the autonomic nervous system	40,41
	Exercise may result in changes in serum osmolality within mucosal tissues, similar to a mechanism that has been implicated in exercise-induced asthma. Hyperosmolality increases basophil histamine release in response to allergens.	42–45
Wheat-dependent FDEIAn specifically	Exercise may induce changes in the processing of specific allergens, leading to increased allergenicity. Many patients with wheat-dependent FDEIAn are sensitized to omega-5 gliadin, and exercise activates intestinal enzyme tissue transglutaminase. This enzyme is capable of binding and aggregating gliadin moieties to form large immunogenic complexes that show increased IgE binding.	46–48

Clinical History

It is critical to confirm that exercise/exertion was associated with every instance of symptoms. For suspected FDEIAn, was there a certain food that was ingested before each episode or is there a food that the patient eats nearly every day (eg, grains)? Did the patient ever have symptoms with exercise first thing in the morning, before eating anything? Did symptoms begin to subside when/if the patient stopped the activity? Have symptoms mostly occurred at certain time of year (peak pollen season) or in certain environmental conditions (high heat and humidity)? Everything the patient ate or drank before each episode should be reviewed (including health drinks, protein bars, or other supplements, which patients often overlook). What medications does the patient take regularly and as needed (especially NSAIDs)? Does the patient have other atopic disorders, especially incompletely controlled allergic rhinitis, asthma, or chronic urticaria? Concomitant uncontrolled allergic disease can lower the threshold for symptoms in some patients.

Physical Examination

No physical findings are unique to patients with EIAn or FDEIAn. Potentially relevant findings include signs of allergic diseases, such as stigmata of longstanding allergic rhinitis. A careful skin examination should be performed to ensure that urticaria pigmentosa, the characteristic skin finding in mastocytosis, is not present. Cardiac examination to exclude abnormal heart sounds or rhythms is appropriate in patients with syncope and near-syncope, as exercise-exacerbated cardiac conditions are in the differential diagnosis.

Laboratory Studies

A baseline serum tryptase level should be measured in all patients. Serum tryptase is normal at baseline in both EIAn and FDEIAn. Elevated values at baseline are suggestive of mast cell disorders. Elevations in serum tryptase or serum or plasma histamine immediately after an episode of symptoms support the diagnosis of anaphylaxis but do not provide information about exercise or food/exercise as the trigger.[57] Data about how often elevations in these mediators are present after episodes of EIAn and FDEIAn are limited to case reports.

Skin Testing or In Vitro Testing

In patients with suspected FDEIAn, skin testing or in vitro testing for food-specific IgE is essential to the evaluation, because sensitization to the precipitating food(s) is usually demonstrable, with rare exceptions.[58] If skin testing with a commercial extract yields negative results, skin testing with fresh food (such as wheat flour paste or the wheat product that the patient ingested before an episode) should be performed, because the use of fresh food appears to be more sensitive.[18,59] For example, in a German series of 17 patients with wheat-dependent FDEIAn, 29% had a positive skin prick test result when tested with a commercial wheat extract, whereas 80% had a positive skin prick test result when tested with a paste of wheat flour.[59]

In a Japanese study of 50 patients with FDEIAn caused by wheat, the sensitivity of the ImmunoCAP (Phadia; Uppsala, Sweden) commercial assay for IgE to recombinant omega-5 gliadin was found to be 80% in patients with positive food/exercise challenges, making this immunoassay more clinically useful than in vitro tests for IgE to wheat (all components), gluten, or other allergens.[60] IgE to omega-5 gliadin may be positive even when an IgE immunoassay to wheat is negative.[61] In patients known to be sensitized to omega-5 gliadin, skin testing with pure gluten flour, which is rich in omega-5 gliadin, appears to be highly sensitive.[18] However, omega-5 gliadin is not the only wheat allergen to be implicated in wheat-dependent FDEIAn, and some patients are sensitized to other wheat allergens.[59]

Although not a routine part of the evaluation, skin testing or in vitro testing for IgE sensitization to environmental allergens is useful in the evaluation of EIAn if specific co-triggers, such as high pollen counts in a patient with concomitant allergic rhinitis or asthma, are suspected. Optimizing the management of coexisting allergic disorders seems to be helpful in reducing the patient's overall reactivity (see later discussion).

Exercise Challenge Testing

A positive exercise challenge (with food for FDEIAn) confirms the diagnosis, but a negative challenge does not reliably exclude the diagnosis for the reasons described in this section. Some centers with experience in EIAn/FDEIAn perform exercise challenges, with and without the culprit food in cases of suspected FDEIAn. There is no established protocol for exercise challenge to evaluate patients for EIAn or FDEIAn, although the

Table 2
Disorders that may be mistaken for EIAn or FDEIAn

Disorder	Can Be Confused With	Features That Help Distinguish Disorder from EIAn or FDEIAn	Helpful Referrals and Testing	Useful References
Cholinergic urticaria	EIAn	Symptoms usually limited to skin but can become systemic. Cholinergic urticaria lesions are small, pinpoint hives on an erythematous skin (vs larger hives with EIAn). Triggered by shifts in body temperature or sweating: occurs during exercise but also during passive changes in body temperature or sweating, such as hot showers, saunas, or strong emotions. Not consistently related to eating or a specific food, although spicy food can be an occasional trigger.	Passive warm water exposure or passive heating and cooling should elicit symptoms of cholinergic urticarial.	49,50
Postural orthostatic tachycardia syndrome	EIAn	Tachycardia develops with change from sitting/lying to standing posture. Symptoms with exercise are common and consistent. Patients may report palpitations, lightheadedness, headache, abdominal discomfort or nausea, fatigue, inappropriate sweating or flushing. However, urticaria, throat tightness, asthmatic symptoms should not be present. Edema may be present, but should be gravitationally dependent.	Cardiology referral, abnormal tilt table testing, abnormal 24-h urine sodium excretion	51
Cardiovascular events	EIAn	Patient may present with flushing, lightheadedness, syncope, tachycardia. However, urticaria, angioedema, throat tightness, and asthmatic symptoms should not be present.	Cardiology referral Holter monitor Stress testing	52

Exercise-induced bronchoconstriction	EIAn	Can mimic EIAn because patient may have chest symptoms, cough, flushing. Patients can report throat tightness and stridor if there is accompanying vocal cord dysfunction. However, urticaria and angioedema should not be present. Symptoms of exercise-induced bronchoconstriction often peak 10–15 min after the completion of exercise.	Response to prophylactic albuterol taken before exercise and other asthma medications. Formal exercise testing with pulmonary function sometimes needed.	53
Exercise-induced gastroesophageal reflux disease (GERD)	FDEIAn	Can mimic EIAn or FDEIAn because patient may have throat symptoms, flushing, and chest symptoms. However, urticaria and angioedema should not be present. Careful history may reveal that patient also has some symptoms of GERD unrelated to exercise.	Gastroenterology referral. Response to H2 antihistamines or proton pump inhibitors.	54
Mast cell disorders • Systemic mastocytosis • Monoclonal mast cell activation syndrome • Mast cell activation syndrome	EIAn or FDEIAn	Symptoms triggered by a variety of situations and not limited to exercise. These include exposure to medications (eg, NSAIDS, narcotics), physical factors other than exercise (massage, extremes of temperature), ingestion of spicy food or alcohol, surgical instrumentation, emotional stress, infections, hymenoptera stings and other toxic exposures. Urticaria pigmentosa (or other less common cutaneous signs of mast cell disease) may be present on skin	Elevated serum tryptase when patient in baseline state. Mutational analysis of KIT showing a codon 816 mutation (eg, Asp816Val), usually in bone marrow or peripheral blood	55,56
Idiopathic anaphylaxis	EIAn or FDEIAn	Not consistently related to exercise (this can be difficult to determine if patient has had just 1 or 2 episodes)		

standard Bruce protocol for stress testing, with the addition of spirometry before and periodically during the procedure, has been used by several groups.[3,25] However, one difficulty surrounding the use of challenges is that symptoms of EIAn and FDEIAn can be difficult to elicit, and studies have reported variable rates of success in eliciting symptoms.[1,3,17,18,25,30,49] Thus, a negative test result does not necessarily exclude FDEIAn. The amount of food, processing, the interval between food ingestion and exercise, and the intensity of the exercise may all be contributing variables.[1,17,18,57] The likelihood of eliciting symptoms at the time of exercise challenge can be increased by administering greater amounts of food, NSAIDs, or alcohol before exercise.[18,60] Challenge procedures are not done at the author's center, largely for reasons of medical legal liability surrounding the deliberate induction of anaphylaxis. If pursued, exercise challenge procedures should be performed by allergy specialists with the expertise, staff, and equipment available to treat anaphylaxis, and informed consent should be obtained from the patient or caregiver.

Food Avoidance as a Diagnostic Tool

Based on the author's experience that FDEIAn is the more common disorder, attacks may be assumed to be food dependent until proven otherwise. The author initially advises avoidance of eating for 4 hours before exercise in nearly all cases. If no further attacks occur, then the period of fasting before exercise can be gradually reduced over time. If symptoms recur as the restrictions are removed, then this provides further useful information, and the evaluation can then focus on the foods that were eaten in those situations. In particular, the patient should be questioned again about snacks, candy, protein bars, and other things they might have eaten that were not part of a formal meal, as patients tend to overlook these items. Also, they may have tolerated a small amount of a certain food on other occasions before exercise, and thus do not think of it as a potential culprit. However, the amount of food can be important in some patients, and a small amount of food may provoke symptoms on one occasion and not another.

DIFFERENTIAL DIAGNOSIS

The differential diagnosis of EIAn and FDEIAn includes several disorders (see **Table 2**).

MANAGEMENT

The management of EIAn and FDEIAn must be individualized for each patient, to some extent, depending on the severity and frequency of symptoms, the importance of food or other co-triggers, and the patient's desire to continue participating in the particular sports or types of exercise that trigger symptoms. Randomized trials of therapies for EIAn or FDEIAn are lacking. The literature is limited to case reports and small series. The authors' approach is described here.

Management of both EIAn and FDEIAn involves the following components:

- Educating the patient about the importance of stopping exercise immediately at the first sign of symptoms
- Preparing the patient to self-administer epinephrine if needed
- Ensuring that future exercise takes place under safe conditions
- Identification and avoidance of causative foods (in FDEIAn)
- Avoidance of co-triggers (eg, NSAIDs, high humidity)
- In some cases, medications to help prevent or reduce symptoms

Management does *not* involve advising the patient to refrain from exercise on a permanent basis. Avoidance of the triggering activity often is prudent in the period between the onset of symptoms and the initial evaluation, but it should not be necessary once the details of the case are understood.

Management of FDEIAn is relatively straightforward in cases in which a specific food can be clearly implicated, because avoidance of that food before exercise is all that is required to prevent attacks. However, even in this situation, there are several issues that may arise (see later discussion).

Patient Education and Access to Epinephrine

Patients must become vigilant for the earliest symptoms of their attacks (usually extreme fatigue, flushing, and pruritus) and must stop exercising immediately when these appear. At the first sign of symptoms, the patient should stop all activity, get an epinephrine autoinjector ready at-hand, and, if lightheaded or dizzy, lie down in a nearby and safe location. If symptoms do not immediately begin to improve, epinephrine should be administered without delay. Some patients additionally carry a dose of orally dissolvable antihistamine, which is helpful for milder symptoms, such as isolated urticaria. However, cessation of exercise is the most important early intervention.

It is helpful to formulate a detailed plan with each patient about how he or she will ensure that medications and a cell phone are always accessible when exercising. In the case of children and adolescents, the parent or caregiver should help with this process. Usually these items can be carried in a small pack worn at the waist. Runners, in particular, are hesitant to carry bulky items, and addressing this issue up front can prevent noncompliance. Such patients often prefer the newer epinephrine auto injectors that are similar in size to cell phones and fit in the arm bands and clothing pockets designed for cell phones. Patients involved in team sports cannot usually have these items on their person, but they should be immediately accessible at the sidelines or held by the coach. Having these items locked in a locker is not adequate.

Other Precautions When Resuming Exercise

- Once evaluation for causative foods and other co-triggers has been completed, patients may resume exercise gradually, starting with a low-level exertion that will probably be tolerated, and gradually to increase their activity over weeks to months.
- Warming up before exercise was identified as helpful in a retrospective series of patients with EIAn.[11] The patient should choose an activity that consistently allows for a warm-up period.
- Patients with EIAn should exercise with a companion or in a supervised setting at all times, at least for the first months after the diagnosis until the physician and patient have a sense for whether the attacks will be controllable. The companion/coach should be educated about the signs and symptoms of anaphylaxis and be capable of administering epinephrine.
- The physician should ask the patient if there are any situations in which he or she would be reluctant to stop exercise. This issue arises with adolescents participating in team sports (eg, competitive cheerleading) in which they are an essential member. In this situation, the patient may be tempted to push through mild symptoms against medical advice for the sake of the team. It is better to avoid these situations by choosing appropriate activities or making a plan in advance for how the patient could be rapidly removed and a substitute put in place.
- As with prevention of anaphylaxis of any etiology, patients should avoid certain medications going forward, such as β-blockers and ACE inhibitors. Medication

lists should be reviewed regularly at follow-up visits to ensure that other providers have not prescribed the same medications. NSAIDs should be avoided for 24 hours before exercise in patients with FDEIAn.[24]

Food Avoidance in Patients with Food-dependent Exercise-induced Anaphylaxis

Patients with FDEIAn should avoid the culprit foods for at least 4 hours before exercise. Exercising in the morning, before eating anything, is a simple way to comply with this restriction. Some patients can restrict the food for fewer hours and others require longer periods (eg, 6 hours).

Avoidance of the culprit food can be difficult in certain scenarios:

- Patients who have symptoms with even mild exertion, such as brisk walking, may have to avoid the culprit food completely, rather than only before exercise. Similarly, children, who run and play unpredictably throughout the day, may need to avoid the culprit food completely.
- Adolescents may need help from parents and clinicians to devise a list of safe foods that they can have on hand, especially for snacking before and during sports practices.

Avoidance of Relevant Co-triggers

- Patients whose attacks follow ingestion of NSAIDs can avoid these agents altogether or at least refrain from exercise for 24 hours after taking one of these medicines.
- Those affected by high humidity or high pollen counts can exercise in an air-conditioned, indoor setting during critical times of year. Allergen immunotherapy can reduce sensitivity to pollen, although this has not been specifically studied in patients with EIAn and concomitant pollen allergy.
- Maximal management of any concomitant allergic disorders, such as allergic rhinitis and asthma, is also helpful.

Preventative Therapies

Prophylactic pharmacotherapy is not needed in cases in which behavior can be modified and co-triggers avoided. However, this is not practical in all cases, and prophylactic pharmacotherapy is sometimes warranted.

Cromolyn Sodium in Food-dependent Exercise-induced Anaphylaxis

Case reports suggest that high-dose cromolyn sodium taken orally before food ingestion can be useful in preventing attack in patients FDEIAn.[16,62–64] The patients in these cases have included children and young adults with FDEIAn who were advised to avoid exercise for 4 hours after eating but found it difficult to comply with this restriction. Oral cromolyn sodium was administered 20 minutes before the midday meal in case there was unexpected exercise in the afternoon.[63] In a report of 2 children, this approach appeared to prevent the children from having symptoms when they did exercise after eating. The children only had symptoms on days when they forgot to take the cromolyn sodium. Over time, both children resumed unrestricted exercise after eating, managing the disorder with cromolyn before the preceding meal.[63]

In 2 case reports of adult patients with wheat-dependent FDEIAn, premedication with cromolyn sodium prevented absorption of wheat allergen into the blood in one patient[64] and prevented an increase in plasma histamine in another.[62] However, in another case report of wheat-dependent FDEIAn, 100 mg of sodium cromoglycate taken 1 hour before food/exercise challenge prevented neither symptoms nor absorption of gliadin into the blood.[65] Of note, the dose used in this report (100 mg) was low for an adult.

Until better data are available, it seems prudent to offer this therapy to patients with a clear warning that the efficacy has not been well defined. It is explained to patients that this approach should NOT be considered a reliable alternative to avoidance of the culprit food but rather an additional protective measure.

Cromolyn sodium comes in an oral formulation (Gastrocrom) in the United States, in ampules of 100 mg/5 mL. The dose used in the reports previously described of children was 100 mg taken before eating. The dose for adults is 200 mg, which is the dose used in the author's practice. We advise patients to take cromolyn sodium in water 30 minutes before any meal that could be followed by exertion and up to four times daily.

H1 Antihistamines

Premedication with H1 antihistamines to prevent ElAn has not been systematically studied. Clinical experience suggests that antihistamines do *not* prevent symptoms, and some clinicians prefer not to initiate antihistamines due to concern for masking early symptoms. However, H1 antihistamine premedication may reduce the severity of episodes in some patients,[10] particularly if they have coexistent allergic rhinitis that is incompletely controlled. Thus, these agents can be prescribed empirically to patients who have not already tried them and discontinued later if there is no apparent benefit after explaining the pros and cons to the patient. The author's approach is to continue antihistamines if the patient presents already taking these medications for other allergic disorders (eg, allergic rhinitis) but to focus on identifying the relevant foods and or other co-triggers, as antihistamines do not seem to have a dramatic impact on ElAn or FDEIAn.

Other Agents

Case reports suggest that misoprostol (a synthetic analogue of prostaglandin E1),[65,66] or omalizumab[67] can be helpful for patients who have not responded to other measures. The author knows of no studies evaluating the use of oral corticosteroids or leukotriene-modifying agents in ElAn or FDEIAn.

PROGNOSIS

Few fatalities are attributed to ElAn or FDEIAn. Literature review found 4 reported fatalities.[68–71] Of these, one had autopsy findings suggesting concomitant bowel ulceration, 2 patients had fatal attacks before the disorder was recognized as exercise related (and both had significant asthma as a comorbidity), and a fourth fatality occurred after ingestion of the known culprit food combined with alcohol, exercise, and no access to epinephrine. Thus, each of these cases had extenuating circumstances.

Fortunately, most patients with ElAn or FDEIAn do well, reporting fewer attacks over time.[11,19] This is likely caused by a combination of recognition of early symptoms, modifications in exercise habits, and avoidance of culprit foods and other co-triggers.

SUMMARY/FUTURE CONSIDERATIONS

ElAn and FDEIAn are uncommon and unpredictable disorders that usually affect otherwise healthy and active individuals. Diagnosis depends heavily on suggestive clinical features and exclusion of other possible disorders. Treatment and prevention are focused on identification of foods and other factors that are relevant for each patient. Important areas for future investigations include standardization of a diagnostic approach (including safe and consistently effective challenge protocols), clarification of the pathogenesis of these disorders, and controlled trials to define the efficacy of pharmacotherapy.

REFERENCES

1. Romano A, Di Fonso M, Giuffreda F, et al. Food-dependent exercise-induced anaphylaxis: clinical and laboratory findings in 54 subjects. Int Arch Allergy Immunol 2001;125:264.
2. Orhan F, Karakas T. Food-dependent exercise-induced anaphylaxis to lentil and anaphylaxis to chickpea in a 17-year-old boy. J Investig Allergol Clin Immunol 2008;18:465.
3. Aihara Y, Takahashi Y, Kotoyori T, et al. Frequency of food-dependent, exercise-induced anaphylaxis in Japanese junior-high-school students. J Allergy Clin Immunol 2001;108:1035.
4. Du Toit G. Food-dependent exercise-induced anaphylaxis in childhood. Pediatr Allergy Immunol 2007;18:455.
5. Barg W, Wolanczyk-Medrala A, Obojski A, et al. Food-dependent exercise-induced anaphylaxis: possible impact of increased basophil histamine releasability in hyperosmolar conditions. J Investig Allergol Clin Immunol 2008;18:312.
6. Beaudouin E, Renaudin JM, Morisset M, et al. Food-dependent exercise-induced anaphylaxis–update and current data. Eur Ann Allergy Clin Immunol 2006;38:45.
7. Longley S, Panush RS. Familial exercise-induced anaphylaxis. Ann Allergy 1987; 58:257.
8. Grant JA, Farnam J, Lord RA, et al. Familial exercise-induced anaphylaxis. Ann Allergy 1985;54:35.
9. Maulitz RM, Pratt DS, Schocket AL. Exercise-induced anaphylactic reaction to shellfish. J Allergy Clin Immunol 1979;63:433.
10. Sheffer AL, Austen KF. Exercise-induced anaphylaxis. J Allergy Clin Immunol 1980;66:106.
11. Shadick NA, Liang MH, Partridge AJ, et al. The natural history of exercise-induced anaphylaxis: survey results from a 10-year follow-up study. J Allergy Clin Immunol 1999;104:123.
12. Pérez-Rangel I, Gonzalo-Garijo MA, Pérez-Calderón R, et al. Wheat-dependent exercise-induced anaphylaxis in elderly patients. Ann Allergy Asthma Immunol 2013;110:121.
13. Wolańczyk-Medrala A, Barg W, Radlińska A, et al. Food-dependent exercise-induced anaphylaxis-sequence of causative factors might be reversed. Ann Agric Environ Med 2010;17:315.
14. Kidd JM 3rd, Cohen SH, Sosman AJ, et al. Food-dependent exercise-induced anaphylaxis. J Allergy Clin Immunol 1983;71:407.
15. Aihara Y, Kotoyori T, Takahashi Y, et al. The necessity for dual food intake to provoke food-dependent exercise-induced anaphylaxis (FEIAn): a case report of FEIAn with simultaneous intake of wheat and umeboshi. J Allergy Clin Immunol 2001;107:1100.
16. Adachi A, Horikawa T, Shimizu H, et al. Soybean beta-conglycinin as the main allergen in a patient with food-dependent exercise-induced anaphylaxis by tofu: food processing alters pepsin resistance. Clin Exp Allergy 2009;39:167.
17. Hanakawa Y, Tohyama M, Shirakata Y, et al. Food-dependent exercise-induced anaphylaxis: a case related to the amount of food allergen ingested. Br J Dermatol 1998;138:898.

18. Brockow K, Kneissl D, Valentini L, et al. Using a gluten oral food challenge protocol to improve diagnosis of wheat-dependent exercise-induced anaphylaxis. J Allergy Clin Immunol 2014.
19. Kano H, Juji F, Shibuya N, et al. Clinical courses of 18 cases with food-dependent exercise-induced anaphylaxis. Arerugi 2000;49:472 [in Japanese].
20. Romano A, Scala E, Rumi G, et al. Lipid transfer proteins: the most frequent sensitizer in Italian subjects with food-dependent exercise-induced anaphylaxis. Clin Exp Allergy 2012;42:1643.
21. Asero R, Mistrello G, Roncarolo D, et al. Exercise-induced egg anaphylaxis. Allergy 1997;52:687.
22. Harada S, Horikawa T, Ashida M, et al. Aspirin enhances the induction of type I allergic symptoms when combined with food and exercise in patients with food-dependent exercise-induced anaphylaxis. Br J Dermatol 2001; 145:336.
23. Matsuo H, Morimoto K, Akaki T, et al. Exercise and aspirin increase levels of circulating gliadin peptides in patients with wheat-dependent exercise-induced anaphylaxis. Clin Exp Allergy 2005;35:461.
24. Fujii H, Kambe N, Fujisawa A, et al. Food-dependent exercise-induced anaphylaxis induced by low dose aspirin therapy. Allergol Int 2008;57:97.
25. Aihara M, Miyazawa M, Osuna H, et al. Food-dependent exercise-induced anaphylaxis: influence of concurrent aspirin administration on skin testing and provocation. Br J Dermatol 2002;146:466.
26. Bito T, Kanda E, Tanaka M, et al. Cows milk-dependent exercise-induced anaphylaxis under the condition of a premenstrual or ovulatory phase following skin sensitization. Allergol Int 2008;57:437.
27. Wade JP, Liang MH, Sheffer AL. Exercise-induced anaphylaxis: epidemiologic observations. Prog Clin Biol Res 1989;297:175.
28. Sheffer AL, Austen KF. Exercise-induced anaphylaxis. J Allergy Clin Immunol 1984;73:699.
29. Lewis J, Lieberman P, Treadwell G, et al. Exercise-induced urticaria, angioedema, and anaphylactoid episodes. J Allergy Clin Immunol 1981;68:432.
30. Sheffer AL, Soter NA, McFadden ER Jr, et al. Exercise-induced anaphylaxis: a distinct form of physical allergy. J Allergy Clin Immunol 1983;71:311.
31. Oyefara BI, Bahna SL. Delayed food-dependent, exercise-induced anaphylaxis. Allergy Asthma Proc 2007;28:64.
32. Schwartz HJ. Elevated serum tryptase in exercise-induced anaphylaxis. J Allergy Clin Immunol 1995;95:917.
33. Casale TB, Bowman S, Kaliner M. Induction of human cutaneous mast cell degranulation by opiates and endogenous opioid peptides: evidence for opiate and nonopiate receptor participation. J Allergy Clin Immunol 1984; 73:775.
34. Lin RY, Barnard M. Skin testing with food, codeine, and histamine in exercise-induced anaphylaxis. Ann Allergy 1993;70:475.
35. Tharp MD, Thirlby R, Sullivan TJ. Gastrin induces histamine release from human cutaneous mast cells. J Allergy Clin Immunol 1984;74:159.
36. Yano H, Kato Y, Matsuda T. Acute exercise induces gastrointestinal leakage of allergen in lysozyme-sensitized mice. Eur J Appl Physiol 2002;87:358.
37. Lichtenberger LM, Zhou Y, Dial EJ, et al. NSAID injury to the gastrointestinal tract: evidence that NSAIDs interact with phospholipids to weaken the hydrophobic surface barrier and induce the formation of unstable pores in membranes. J Pharm Pharmacol 2006;58:1421.

38. Cooper DM, Radom-Aizik S, Schwindt C, et al. Dangerous exercise: lessons learned from dysregulated inflammatory responses to physical activity. J Appl Physiol (1985) 2007;103:700.
39. Robson-Ansley P, Toit GD. Pathophysiology, diagnosis and management of exercise-induced anaphylaxis. Curr Opin Allergy Clin Immunol 2010;10:312.
40. Fukutomi O, Kondo N, Agata H, et al. Abnormal responses of the autonomic nervous system in food-dependent exercise-induced anaphylaxis. Ann Allergy 1992; 68:438.
41. Kato Y, Nagai A, Saito M, et al. Food-dependent exercise-induced anaphylaxis with a high level of plasma noradrenaline. J Dermatol 2007;34:110.
42. Anderson SD, Daviskas E. The mechanism of exercise-induced asthma is.... J Allergy Clin Immunol 2000;106:453.
43. Eggleston PA, Kagey-Sobotka A, Schleimer RP, et al. Interaction between hyperosmolar and IgE-mediated histamine release from basophils and mast cells. Am Rev Respir Dis 1984;130:86.
44. Nielsen BW, Bjerke T, Damsgaard TM, et al. Hyperosmolarity selectively enhances IgE-receptor-mediated histamine release from human basophils. Agents Actions 1992;35:170.
45. Stellato C, de Crescenzo G, Patella V, et al. Human basophil/mast cell releasability. XI. Heterogeneity of the effects of contrast media on mediator release. J Allergy Clin Immunol 1996;97:838.
46. Palosuo K, Alenius H, Varjonen E, et al. A novel wheat gliadin as a cause of exercise-induced anaphylaxis. J Allergy Clin Immunol 1999;103:912.
47. Daengsuwan T, Palosuo K, Phankingthongkum S, et al. IgE antibodies to omega-5 gliadin in children with wheat-induced anaphylaxis. Allergy 2005; 60:506.
48. Palosuo K, Varjonen E, Nurkkala J, et al. Transglutaminase-mediated cross-linking of a peptic fraction of omega-5 gliadin enhances IgE reactivity in wheat-dependent, exercise-induced anaphylaxis. J Allergy Clin Immunol 2003;111:1386.
49. Romano A, Di Fonso M, Giuffreda F, et al. Diagnostic work-up for food-dependent, exercise-induced anaphylaxis. Allergy 1995;50:817.
50. Kaplan AP, Natbony SF, Tawil AP, et al. Exercise-induced anaphylaxis as a manifestation of cholinergic urticaria. J Allergy Clin Immunol 1981;68:319.
51. Altrichter S, Salow J, Ardelean E, et al. Development of a standardized pulse-controlled ergometry test for diagnosing and investigating cholinergic urticaria. J Dermatol Sci 2014;75:88.
52. Behera SK, Pattnaik T, Luke A. Practical recommendations and perspectives on cardiac screening for healthy pediatric athletes. Curr Sports Med Rep 2011; 10(2):90–8.
53. Johnson JN, Mack KJ, Kuntz NL, et al. Postural orthostatic tachycardia syndrome: a clinical review. Pediatr Neurol 2010;42:77.
54. Parsons JP, Hallstrand TS, Mastronarde JG, et al. An official American Thoracic Society clinical practice guideline: exercise-induced bronchoconstriction. Am J Respir Crit Care Med 2013;187:1016.
55. Jozkow P, Wasko-Czopnik D, Medras M, et al. Gastroesophageal reflux disease and physical activity. Sports Med 2006;36:385.
56. Valent P. Mast cell activation syndromes. Allergy 2013;68:417.
57. Loibl M, Schwarz S, Ring J, et al. Definition of an exercise intensity threshold in a challenge test to diagnose food-dependent exercise-induced anaphylaxis. Allergy 2009;64:1560.

58. Kleiman J, Ben-Shoshan M. Food-dependent exercise-induced anaphylaxis with negative allergy testing. BMJ Case Rep 2014;2014.
59. Hofmann SC, Fischer J, Eriksson C, et al. IgE detection to $\alpha/\beta/\gamma$-gliadin and its clinical relevance in wheat-dependent exercise-induced anaphylaxis. Allergy 2012;67:1457.
60. Matsuo H, Dahlström J, Tanaka A, et al. Sensitivity and specificity of recombinant omega-5 gliadin-specific IgE measurement for the diagnosis of wheat-dependent exercise-induced anaphylaxis. Allergy 2008;63:233.
61. Park HJ, Kim JH, Kim JE, et al. Diagnostic value of the serum-specific IgE ratio of ω-5 gliadin to wheat in adult patients with wheat-induced anaphylaxis. Int Arch Allergy Immunol 2012;157:147.
62. Juji F, Suko M. Effectiveness of disodium cromoglycate in food-dependent, exercise-induced anaphylaxis: a case report. Ann Allergy 1994;72:452.
63. Sugimura T, Tananari Y, Ozaki Y, et al. Effect of oral sodium cromoglycate in 2 children with food-dependent exercise-induced anaphylaxis (FDEIA). Clin Pediatr (Phila) 2009;48:945.
64. Ueno M, Adachi A, Shimoura S, et al. A case of wheat-dependent exercise-induced anaphylaxis controlled by sodium chromoglycate, but not controlled by misoprostol. J Environ Dermatol Cutan Allergol 2008;2:118.
65. Takahashi A, Nakajima K, Ikeda M, et al. Pre-treatment with misoprostol prevents food-dependent exercise-induced anaphylaxis (FDEIA). Int J Dermatol 2011;50:237.
66. Inoue Y, Adachi A, Ueno M, et al. The inhibition effect of a synthetic analogue of prostaglandin E1 to the provocation by aspirin in the patients of WDEIA. Arerugi 2009;58:1418 [in Japanese].
67. Bray SM, Fajt ML, Petrov AA. Successful treatment of exercise-induced anaphylaxis with omalizumab. Ann Allergy Asthma Immunol 2012;109:281.
68. Ausdenmoore RW. Fatality in a teenager secondary to exercise-induced anaphylaxis. Pediatr Asthma Allergy Immunol 1991;5:21.
69. Drouet M, Sabbah A, Le Sellin J, et al. Fatal anaphylaxis after eating wild boar meat in a patient with pork-cat syndrome. Allerg Immunol (Paris) 2001;33:163 [in French].
70. Flannagan LM, Wolf BC. Sudden death associated with food and exercise. J Forensic Sci 2004;49:543.
71. Noma T, Yoshizawa I, Ogawa N, et al. Fatal buckwheat dependent exercised-induced anaphylaxis. Asian Pac J Allergy Immunol 2001;19:283.

Mast Cell Activation Syndromes Presenting as Anaphylaxis

Cem Akin, MD, PhD

KEYWORDS

- Anaphylaxis • Mastocytosis • Mast cell activation syndrome • Mast cells • Tryptase

KEY POINTS

- Clonal mast cell disease should be suspected in patients presenting with recurrent hypotensive syncopal or near-syncopal episodes without urticaria or angioedema.
- Patients with severe systemic reactions to hymenoptera and elevated baseline tryptase levels should be investigated for presence of mastocytosis. These patients should be considered for life-long venom immunotherapy if evidence for IgE-mediated venom sensitization is found.
- Mast cell activation syndrome is a multisystem disorder with specific diagnostic criteria.
- Documentation of elevated mast cell mediator levels during episodes is critical to diagnosis because some symptoms may not be specific to mast cell activation.

Anaphylaxis is the end result of massive systemic mast cell activation. Physiologic mast cell activation is thought to be beneficial in innate immunity against microorganisms, wound healing, regulation of coagulation, and neutralization of venoms.[1] Pathologic mast cell activation on the other hand is a disproportionate display of mast cell activity often in response to an otherwise harmless trigger. Pathologic mast cell activation may accompany primary disorders of mast cells or may occur in response to a trigger such as an allergen. Sometimes, no recognizable provoking factors for mast cell activation can be elicited.

A specific disorder of mast cells presenting with recurrent episodic mast cell activation has been suggested in the literature for decades; however, diagnostic criteria have been proposed only recently.[2] This disorder, also termed mast cell activation syndrome (MCAS), has many overlapping characteristics with idiopathic anaphylaxis (IA), although MCAS episodes may not always have the full clinical picture of anaphylaxis. This article first discusses the global classification of mast cell disorders, then provides clinical features and diagnostic workup for each category.

Disclosure: Consultancy agreements with Novartis, Patara Pharma, and Blueprint Medicines. Department of Medicine, Division of Rheumatology, Immunology and Allergy, Mastocytosis Center, Brigham and Women's Hospital, Harvard Medical School, One Jimmy Fund Way, Room 616D Boston, MA 02115, USA
E-mail address: cakin@partners.org

Immunol Allergy Clin N Am 35 (2015) 277–285
http://dx.doi.org/10.1016/j.iac.2015.01.010
immunology.theclinics.com

GLOBAL CLASSIFICATION OF MAST CELL DISORDERS

Mast cell disorders can be broadly divided into those involving proliferation and those involving activation, often with a substantial overlap. Most patients with a proliferative mast cell disease such as mastocytosis come to clinical attention because of symptoms caused by mast cell activation.[3] Akin and colleagues[2] recently proposed a global classification scheme for disorders associated with mast cell activation based on whether the mast cells have a primary genetic defect or are simply reacting to an exogenous trigger (**Box 1**).

PRIMARY (CLONAL) MAST CELL DISORDERS

Primary (clonal) mast cell disorder includes mastocytosis and its limited variant monoclonal mast cell activation syndrome (MMAS). These disorders are associated with clonal expansion of mast cells carrying genetic defects in the receptor tyrosine kinase c-kit (most often D816V point mutation). Mastocytosis is characterized by pathologic accumulation of mast cells in various tissues, such as skin and bone marrow, and has a strong proliferative feature in which the proliferative component and mast cell burden in MMAS are more subtle.[4] D816V c-kit mutation is a gain-of-function mutation that has shown to be involved in growth factor independence of hematopoietic cell lines, protection from apoptosis, and enhancement of mast cell chemotaxis.[5] There is a complex interplay between the wild-type and mutated KIT product in the cell. The mutated KIT is primarily located intracellularly, whereas the wild-type KIT is displayed on the cell surface.[6] Wild-type KIT is linked by its ligand stem cell factor, which results in dimerization and autophosphorylation of the receptor. D816V-mutated KIT is constitutively active. Whether this activation is directly involved in reduced mast cell activation threshold is not known. One in vitro model based on

---

Box 1
Global classification of disorders associated with mast cell activation

Primary

  Mastocytosis

  Monoclonal mast cell activation syndrome

Secondary

  IgE-mediated

  Non–IgE-mediated

    Physical

    Associated with inflammatory, infectious, or neoplastic disorders

    Direct mast cell activation

    Chronic autoimmune urticaria

Idiopathic

  Idiopathic anaphylaxis

  Idiopathic urticaria and or angioedema

  Mast cell activation syndrome

Adapted from Akin C, Valent P, Metcalfe DD. Mast cell activation syndrome: proposed diagnostic criteria. J Allergy Clin Immunol 2010;126:1099.

overexpression of the mutated KIT in a mast cell line was unable to show enhancement of IgE-mediated mast cell degranulation; however, the extent of this model as an accurate representation of the in vivo environment in mastocytosis is not known.[7]

Mastocytosis can be divided into cutaneous and systemic forms. Cutaneous mastocytosis is the main form of disease in children and is characterized by urticaria pigmentosa or mastocytoma skin lesions without bone marrow or internal organ involvement.[8] There is a rare form of disease involving the whole skin without distinct lesions termed diffuse cutaneous mastocytosis. Cutaneous mastocytosis should be differentiated from urticaria pigmentosa in adults (or mastocytosis in the skin) that often accompanies systemic mastocytosis. Systemic mastocytosis is diagnosed according to the World Health Organization (WHO) criteria, which consist of 1 major and 4 minor criteria.[9] The single major and at least 1 minor, or 3 minor criteria alone, are needed to establish the diagnosis. The major criterion is presence of multifocal compact aggregates of mast cells in tissue biopsies other than skin. The best method to visualize the mast cells is the immunohistochemical stain for tryptase because no other cell stains positively for tryptase (although basophils and myeloid progenitors also contain low levels.) The minor criteria include a serum baseline tryptase level of greater than 20 ng/mL, morphologic abnormalities in mast cells (such as spindle shapes instead of the normal round shape), aberrant CD25 expression by mast cells, and c-kit D816V mutation in peripheral blood or lesional tissue. CD25 expression and c-kit mutation are clonal markers that are not present in clinical samples in which a mild increase in normal mast cell numbers can be seen in reaction to another ongoing inflammatory or neoplastic process (reactive mast cell hyperplasia). Reactive mast cell hyperplasia is thought to reflect a physiologic response of normally produced mast cells to migrate to areas of inflammation such as gut in inflammatory bowel disease, skin in psoriasis, or synovium in rheumatoid arthritis. Mast cells in these conditions may contribute to disease symptoms such as itching or tissue remodeling but do not initiate the pathologic process.

A false-negative result for D816V c-kit mutation is a common clinical problem.[10] This is because the mutation is somatic and is concentrated in tissues with high numbers of pathologic mast cells. Therefore, peripheral blood (and even lesional tissue in cases with low mast cell burden) may not have enough copies of the mutated gene to yield a positive result, especially if a low-sensitive technique such as sequencing is used. A very sensitive method has recently been described that detects an allelic frequency of down to 0.03%; however, the methods to detect the c-kit mutation have not been standardized across laboratories.[11] Aberrant mast cell CD25 expression correlates well with D816V mutation.[12] CD25 can be detected by flow cytometry of the bone marrow aspirate or by immunohistochemistry of the biopsy tissue. Because mast cells are rare events in bone marrow aspirates, at least 500,000 cells should be acquired to be able to analyze the mast cells by flow cytometry. High autofluorescence of atypical mast cells also complicates interpretation of the data. CD25 immunohistochemistry can be performed in routinely processed, paraffin-embedded tissue, including archival specimens, and may be the most easily accessible diagnostic marker in general pathology laboratories.[13] The most common tissue used for the diagnosis of mastocytosis is bone marrow, although some cases were initially diagnosed on gastrointestinal (GI) biopsies. Mast cells in mastocytosis GI biopsies form a typical band in the subepithelial area, generally exceed 100 per high power field,[14] and CD25 staining is positive. Interestingly, tryptase seems to be variably expressed in GI mast cells in mastocytosis and, therefore, CD117 staining should be done in suspected cases.

Monoclonal mast cell activation is a more recently introduced term to designate cases in which patients who, on presentation, have detectable D816V c-kit mutation or CD25+ mast cells but do not meet the full WHO diagnostic criteria.[15,16] These patients present with symptoms of mast cell activation but lack skin lesions of urticaria pigmentosa. Tryptase levels may be normal or mildly elevated and may not exceed 20 ng/mL at baseline. It is not known if all patients with MMAS will eventually develop systemic mastocytosis or whether some may have a self-limited course with eventual resolution; however, limited data suggest that some patients remain in this state for many years without a cumulative increase in mast cell burden.

ANAPHYLAXIS IN CLONAL MAST CELL DISEASE

It has been clearly established that the incidence of anaphylaxis is increased in mastocytosis. Several reports from Europe and the United States point to an average incidence of 30% lifetime risk of anaphylaxis in patients with mastocytosis.[17–19] Anaphylaxis in mastocytosis and MMAS may be due to an IgE-mediated event, may be caused by direct mast cell activation, or may have no clear triggers. Among IgE-mediated triggers, the risk of hymenoptera anaphylaxis is the best studied. It seems that elevated tryptase levels correlate with the severity of systemic reactions to hymenoptera stings (as well as systemic reactions to venom immunotherapy) regardless of the diagnosis of mastocytosis.[20] One large study from Italy found that approximately 10% of subjects with systemic reactions to hymenoptera had elevated tryptase levels of greater than 11.4 ng/mL.[21] Most of these subjects had mastocytosis or MMAS diagnosed by bone marrow biopsies. In some patients, hymenoptera anaphylaxis may be the only clinical symptom that may lead to the diagnosis of mastocytosis. Most of these patients have evidence of venom-specific IgE on blood or skin tests although specific IgE levels may be lower compared with the nonmastocytosis venom allergic population, possibly due to the adsorption of IgE onto the increased numbers of mast cells, making it less available to be detected in the serum. Venom immunotherapy is indicated indefinitely in this patient population. It is important to establish the diagnosis correctly because fatalities due to insect stings have been reported in patients with mastocytosis.[22,23] IgE-mediated anaphylaxis to drugs and foods are not well studied in mastocytosis. There are occasional case reports of patients with allergy to foods or preservatives.[24] Some patients with mastocytosis have flushing and gastrointestinal symptoms triggered by spicy foods and alcohol; however, these symptoms rarely progress to anaphylaxis. However, cumulative clinical experience suggests that the incidence of IgE-mediated food allergy is not greater in mastocytosis patients compared with the general population. Likewise, it is not known whether the incidence of IgE-mediated drug allergy is increased in mastocytosis.[25] Experience suggests some patients may be at risk for severe non IgE-mediated reactions, such as those experienced with nonsteroidal anti-inflammatory drugs, or with perioperative muscle relaxants. Premedication regimens and a list of perioperative drugs with lower intrinsic mast cell activation properties to be used in anesthesia have been proposed.[26] The incidence of mastocytosis in patients formerly diagnosed with IA is also increased. Akin and colleagues[15] reported that 5 out of 12 patients with IA carried clonal mast cell markers. These findings have been confirmed in larger series from Europe.[27,28]

Symptoms of anaphylaxis experienced in patients with clonal mast cell disease seem to be distinct. It is rare for patients with mastocytosis to experience urticaria or angioedema as the main symptom of mastocytosis, whereas hypotension, syncope, and near syncope are common.[28] This can be a helpful feature in deciding which patients may need further diagnostic workup for mastocytosis. The Spanish Network for Mastocytosis (REMA) reported that male gender, baseline tryptase greater than 25 ng/mL, absence of urticaria, and presence of hypotension were all associated with a pretest possibility of mastocytosis and have published a score based on these parameters.[28]

Because diagnosis of mastocytosis requires a tissue biopsy, it may be challenging to decide when to aggressively pursue a diagnosis. One study from Holland found that increased levels of the histamine metabolites methylimidazole acetic acid (MIMA) and N-methylhistamine in the urine were a good predictor of mastocytosis when combined with a baseline tryptase level greater than 10 ng/mL.[29] MIMA measurements are not available commercially in the United States but N-methylhistamine is available commercially as a validated mast cell activation marker. Taken together, the author recommends the following evidence-based guidelines in patients presenting with anaphylaxis for referral for a bone marrow biopsy:

1. Adult patients with urticaria pigmentosa
2. Patients with a baseline tryptase of greater than 25 ng/mL if no evidence of urticaria pigmentosa
3. Patients presenting with recurrent hypotensive syncopal or near-syncopal episodes rather than urticaria or angioedema as the main feature of anaphylaxis, regardless of tryptase levels
4. Patients with elevated tryptase (>11.4 ng/mL) and a history of hymenoptera venom anaphylaxis or elevated urinary histamine metabolites
5. Patients with REMA score[28] of less than or equal to 2

MAST CELL ACTIVATION SYNDROME

The presence of a disorder that is distinct from mastocytosis and is characterized by recurrent mast cell activation episodes has been considered for many years and diagnostic criteria have been recently proposed (**Box 2**).[2,30] Because of the nonspecific nature of many symptoms experienced in a mast cell activation episode and the lack of histopathologic findings, it is important to objectively document a marker of mast cell activation during a symptomatic state. The serum marker that is most specific for mast cell activation is tryptase. Tryptase should be measured in serum or plasma within 4 hours of the suspected event. A suggested meaningful increase is $x + 0.2x + 2$ in which x is the baseline tryptase.[30] Thus, a case in which a patient has a baseline tryptase of 5 ng/mL and an increase of greater than 8 ng/mL during a symptomatic period is suggestive of mast cell activation. Also, 24-hour urinary N-methylhistamine, prostaglandin (PG) D2 (PGD2), or 11-bPGF2α levels correlate

---

Box 2
Proposed diagnostic criteria for mast cell activation syndrome (all 3 must be present)

1. Episodic recurrent symptoms consistent with mast cell activation in more than 1 organ system (skin, GI, cardiovascular, respiratory, nasoocular)

2. Decrease in frequency or severity of symptoms in response to mast cell mediator therapy (H1 and H2 antihistamines, leukotrienes, cromolyn, glucocorticoids)

3. Documentation of increased mast cell activation products above baseline in at least 2 symptomatic episodes (tryptase is the preferred marker; urinary histamine metabolites and PGD2 or 11-b-PGF2α are less specific)

Adapted from Akin C, Valent P, Metcalfe DD. Mast cell activation syndrome: proposed diagnostic criteria. J Allergy Clin Immunol 2010;126:1099.

with mast cell activation when the collection period covers or starts immediately after a symptomatic period. However, specific cutoff limits and the specificity of these markers for mast cell activation have not been established. For example, PGD2 may also be produced by activated eosinophils.[31]

Akin and colleagues[2] initially proposed the term MCAS to designate an idiopathic systemic syndrome presenting with multisystem mast cell activation symptoms documented by increased mast cell mediator levels during attacks, which was distinct from clonal and IgE-mediated disorders. Subsequently, experts at an international conference adopted the diagnostic criteria; however, they proposed that the term be used regardless of presence of a clonal or IgE-mediated disorder.[30] Thus, a patient presenting with mast cell activation symptoms would be first evaluated for presence of MCAS criteria, then be classified into primary, secondary, or idiopathic categories, therefore expanding the scope of the syndrome. This is an area that still lacks universal consensus and, in practice, most clinicians would reserve the term for patients in whom no clear cause for episodes is found.

The clinical overlap between MCAS and IA is also significant. Some experts propose replacing the term IA with MCAS because the latter is a more mechanistic and inclusive terminology because, in patients with IA, not all episodes may rise to the severity of anaphylaxis, especially in those who are on maintenance antihistamine or disease-modifying therapy.

Table 1 provides a comparison of the most pertinent clinical features of mastocytosis and idiopathic MCAS.

MANAGEMENT OF RECURRENT ANAPHYLAXIS ASSOCIATED WITH MAST CELL ACTIVATION SYNDROME

In patients with recurrent anaphylaxis associated with MCAS, the most important step is to clarify if the patient has a clonal, an IgE-mediated, or an idiopathic mast cell disorder. Management of IgE-mediated disorders relies heavily on trigger avoidance, availability of multiple doses of self-injected epinephrine, and desensitization in certain circumstances such as with venom anaphylaxis. Patients with clonal and idiopathic MCAS are generally

Table 1
Comparison of clinicopathologic features of mastocytosis and idiopathic mast cell activation syndrome

Clinicopathologic Feature	Mastocytosis	MCAS
Urticaria and angioedema	Rare	Often present
Hypotensive episodes	Common	May be present
Urticaria pigmentosa	Often present	Absent
Serum baseline tryptase	Often >20 ng/mL	Often <20 ng/mL
Tryptase during the event	Elevated	Elevated
CD25+ mast cells	Yes	No
c-kit D816V mutation	Yes	No
Mast cell clustering in tissue biopsies	Yes, particularly around blood vessels	No, or minimal, not exceeding 2–3 cells
Mast cell shape in bone marrow	Spindled	Round and fully granulated
Urinary mast cell mediators	Elevated	Elevated
Response to H1 antihistamines	Yes	Yes

placed on a maintenance H1-antihistamine therapy (once or twice daily long-acting antihistamine). Siebenhaar and colleagues[32] recommend a stepwise approach in which additional drugs, including H2 antihistamines, antileukotrienes, oral cromolyn, and steroids, are added in unresponsive patients. It is the author's experience that patients with idiopathic MCAS respond similarly to treatment options suggested for IA, including ketotifen,[33] whereas this drug is generally not superior to conventional antihistamines in patients with clonal mast cell disease.[34] Aspirin therapy has been reported beneficial in patients with MCAS who have elevated urinary PG levels.[35] Omalizumab has shown beneficial in suppressing mast cell activation episodes in all clinical subtypes of MCAS, although exact mechanism of action is unknown.[36–38] Patients with clonal mast cell disease who are not responsive to the symptomatic management and who continue to have life-threatening symptoms may be candidates for mast cell cytoreductive therapy, such as interferon-alpha, cladribine, or tyrosine kinase inhibitors.[39] Mast cell clonality should be clearly established before considering cytoreductive therapy and the risks and the benefits of the particular drugs should be carefully discussed with the patient, including the possible investigational nature of the proposed therapy.

FUTURE DIRECTIONS

Despite increased awareness and recognition of MCAS in the last decade, much remains to be elucidated regarding its pathogenesis, disease markers, and treatment. Prospective multicenter trials are needed to validate the proposed diagnostic criteria and identify patient subgroups that may respond differently to therapy. The incidence and subtypes of MCAS in the pediatric population have not been systematically investigated. Although tryptase is the most specific marker for mast cell activation, it has to be checked within a few hours after the episode and may not be elevated in all patients with anaphylaxis. The specificity of urinary PGF2 is not known. Therefore, identification of additional markers of mast cell activation and anaphylaxis would facilitate the diagnosis of MCAS. Finally, development of new drugs targeting intracellular mast cell activation mechanisms and mediators, as well as mast cell survival, is needed. All of these efforts should benefit from basic mechanistic human mast cell research, although they are hampered to a certain degree by the difficulty in obtaining ex vivo human mast cells and the time and cost involved in generating human mast cell cultures. A variety of human mast cell lines, including HMC-1,[40] LAD2,[41] and ROSA,[7] each with its own advantages and shortfalls have been established that could complement these efforts.

REFERENCES

1. Reber LL, Marichal T, Galli SJ. New models for analyzing mast cell functions in vivo. Trends Immunol 2012;12:613.
2. Akin C, Valent P, Metcalfe DD. Mast cell activation syndrome: proposed diagnostic criteria. J Allergy Clin Immunol 2010;126:1099.
3. Jennings S, Russell N, Jennings B, et al. The Mastocytosis Society survey on mast cell disorders: patient experiences and perceptions. J Allergy Clin Immunol Pract 2014;2:70.
4. Akin C, Valent P. Diagnostic criteria and classification of mastocytosis in 2014. Immunol Allergy Clin North Am 2014;34:207.
5. Jensen BM, Metcalfe DD, Gilfillan AM. Targeting kit activation: a potential therapeutic approach in the treatment of allergic inflammation. Inflamm Allergy Drug Targets 2007;6:57.

6. Bougherara H, Subra F, Crépin R, et al. The aberrant localization of oncogenic kit tyrosine kinase receptor mutants is reversed on specific inhibitory treatment. Mol Cancer Res 2009;7:1525.
7. Saleh R, Wedeh G, Herrmann H, et al. A new human mast cell line expressing a functional IgE receptor converts to tumorigenic growth by KIT D816V transfection. Blood 2014;124:111.
8. Fried AJ, Akin C. Primary mast cell disorders in children. Curr Allergy Asthma Rep 2013;13:693.
9. Valent P, Horny HP, Escribano L, et al. Diagnostic criteria and classification of mastocytosis: a consensus proposal. Leuk Res 2001;25:603.
10. Akin C. Molecular diagnosis of mast cell disorders: a paper from the 2005 William Beaumont Hospital Symposium on Molecular Pathology. J Mol Diagn 2006;8:412.
11. Kristensen T, Vestergaard H, Møller MB. Improved detection of the KIT D816V mutation in patients with systemic mastocytosis using a quantitative and highly sensitive real-time qPCR assay. J Mol Diagn 2011;13:180.
12. Teodosio C, García-Montero AC, Jara-Acevedo M, et al. An immature immunophenotype of bone marrow mast cells predicts for multilineage D816V KIT mutation in systemic mastocytosis. Leukemia 2012;26:951.
13. Sotlar K, Horny HP, Simonitsch I, et al. CD25 indicates the neoplastic phenotype of mast cells: a novel immunohistochemical marker for the diagnosis of systemic mastocytosis (SM) in routinely processed bone marrow biopsy specimens. Am J Surg Pathol 2004;28:1319.
14. Doyle LA, Sepehr GJ, Hamilton MJ, et al. A clinicopathologic study of 24 cases of systemic mastocytosis involving the gastrointestinal tract and assessment of mucosal mast cell density in irritable bowel syndrome and asymptomatic patients. Am J Surg Pathol 2014;38:832.
15. Akin C, Scott LM, Kocabas CN, et al. Demonstration of an aberrant mast-cell population with clonal markers in a subset of patients with "idiopathic" anaphylaxis. Blood 2007;110:2331.
16. Sonneck K, Florian S, Müllauer L, et al. Diagnostic and subdiagnostic accumulation of mast cells in the bone marrow of patients with anaphylaxis: monoclonal mast cell activation syndrome. Int Arch Allergy Immunol 2007;142:158.
17. Greenhawt M, Akin C. Mastocytosis and allergy. Curr Opin Allergy Clin Immunol 2007;7:387.
18. Brockow K, Jofer C, Behrendt H, et al. Anaphylaxis in patients with mastocytosis: a study on history, clinical features and risk factors in 120 patients. Allergy 2008;63:226.
19. Matito A, Alvarez-Twose I, Morgado JM, et al. Anaphylaxis as a clinical manifestation of clonal mast cell disorders. Curr Allergy Asthma Rep 2014;14:450.
20. Ruëff F, Przybilla B, Biló MB, et al. Predictors of severe systemic anaphylactic reactions in patients with Hymenoptera venom allergy: importance of baseline serum tryptase-a study of the European Academy of Allergology and Clinical Immunology Interest Group on Insect Venom Hypersensitivity. J Allergy Clin Immunol 2009;124:1047.
21. Bonadonna P, Perbellini O, Passalacqua G, et al. Clonal mast cell disorders in patients with systemic reactions to Hymenoptera stings and increased serum tryptase levels. J Allergy Clin Immunol 2009;123:680.
22. Wagner N, Fritze D, Przybilla B, et al. Fatal anaphylactic sting reaction in a patient with mastocytosis. Int Arch Allergy Immunol 2008;146:162.
23. Oude Elberink JN, de Monchy JG, Kors JW, et al. Fatal anaphylaxis after a yellow jacket sting, despite venom immunotherapy, in two patients with mastocytosis. J Allergy Clin Immunol 1997;99:153.

24. Cifuentes L, Ring J, Brockow K. Clonal mast cell activation syndrome with anaphylaxis to sulfites. Int Arch Allergy Immunol 2013;162:94.
25. Brockow K, Bonadonna P. Drug allergy in mast cell disease. Curr Opin Allergy Clin Immunol 2012;12:354.
26. Dewachter P, Castells MC, Hepner DL, et al. Perioperative management of patients with mastocytosis. Anesthesiology 2014;120:753.
27. Gülen T, Hägglund H, Dahlén B, et al. High prevalence of anaphylaxis in patients with systemic mastocytosis - a single-centre experience. Clin Exp Allergy 2014; 44:121.
28. Alvarez-Twose I, González de Olano D, Sánchez-Muñoz L, et al. Clinical, biological, and molecular characteristics of clonal mast cell disorders presenting with systemic mast cell activation symptoms. J Allergy Clin Immunol 2010;125:1269.
29. van Doormaal JJ, van der Veer E, van Voorst Vader PC, et al. Tryptase and histamine metabolites as diagnostic indicators of indolent systemic mastocytosis without skin lesions. Allergy 2012;67:683.
30. Valent P, Akin C, Arock M, et al. Definitions, criteria and global classification of mast cell disorders with special reference to mast cell activation syndromes: a consensus proposal. Int Arch Allergy Immunol 2012;157:215.
31. Luna-Gomes T, Magalhães KG, Mesquita-Santos FP, et al. Eosinophils as a novel cell source of prostaglandin D2: autocrine role in allergic inflammation. J Immunol 2011;187:6518.
32. Siebenhaar F, Akin C, Bindslev-Jensen C, et al. Treatment strategies in mastocytosis. Immunol Allergy Clin North Am 2014;34:433.
33. Ditto AM, Harris KE, Krasnick J, et al. Idiopathic anaphylaxis: a series of 335 cases. Ann Allergy Asthma Immunol 1996;77:285.
34. Kettelhut BV, Berkebile C, Bradley D, et al. A double-blind, placebo-controlled, crossover trial of ketotifen versus hydroxyzine in the treatment of pediatric mastocytosis. J Allergy Clin Immunol 1989;83:866.
35. Ravi A, Butterfield J, Weiler CR. Mast cell activation syndrome: improved identification by combined determinations of serum tryptase and 24-hour urine 11β-prostaglandin2α. J Allergy Clin Immunol Pract 2014;2:775.
36. Carter MC, Robyn JA, Bressler PB, et al. Omalizumab for the treatment of unprovoked anaphylaxis in patients with systemic mastocytosis. J Allergy Clin Immunol 2007;119:1550.
37. Sokol KC, Ghazi A, Kelly BC, et al. Omalizumab as a desensitizing agent and treatment in mastocytosis: a review of the literature and case report. J Allergy Clin Immunol Pract 2014;2:266.
38. Bell MC, Jackson DJ. Prevention of anaphylaxis related to mast cell activation syndrome with omalizumab. Ann Allergy Asthma Immunol 2012;108:383.
39. Valent P, Sperr WR, Akin C. How I treat patients with advanced systemic mastocytosis. Blood 2010;116:5812.
40. Butterfield JH, Weiler D, Dewald G, et al. Establishment of an immature mast cell line from a patient with mast cell leukemia. Leuk Res 1988;12:345.
41. Kirshenbaum AS, Akin C, Wu Y, et al. Characterization of novel stem cell factor responsive human mast cell lines LAD 1 and 2 established from a patient with mast cell sarcoma/leukemia; activation following aggregation of FcepsilonRI or FcgammaRI. Leuk Res 2003;27:677.

Anaphylaxis to Insect Stings

David B.K. Golden, MD

KEYWORDS

- Anaphylaxis • Venom • Insect sting • Hymenoptera • Immunotherapy
- Diagnostic tests • Mastocytosis

KEY POINTS

- Anaphylaxis to insect stings occurs in 3% of adults and less than 1% of children.
- Anaphylaxis to insect stings is generally more benign in children, but severe reactions can be associated with sustained risk for decades.
- Diagnostic tests can identify the presence of sensitization to insect venom but are poor predictors of sting anaphylaxis.
- There is a specific association between insect-sting anaphylaxis and mastocytosis, particularly when there is hypotension during the reaction.
- Venom immunotherapy is highly effective in preventing sting anaphylaxis, and leads to lasting tolerance in most patients who are treated for 5 years.

INTRODUCTION

Stinging insects of the order Hymenoptera can cause systemic allergic reactions, including anaphylaxis, but such reactions are rare with biting insects. This article describes the clinical patterns and treatment of anaphylaxis to insect stings, and how they may resemble or differ from other causes of anaphylaxis.

CLINICAL FEATURES

Transient pain, itching, and swelling are normal responses to stings, but allergic reactions can cause more severe local reactions or generalized systemic reactions. Large local sting reactions cause delayed and prolonged local inflammation increasing over 24 to 48 hours and resolving in 3 to 10 days. These reactions resemble late-phase inflammatory reactions that are immunoglobulin E (IgE) dependent. Most patients with large local reactions have detectable venom-specific IgE.[1]

Conflicts of interest: Honoraria/speakers bureau for Genentech; consultant for Stallergenes; research grant/clinical trial for Siemens and Genentech.
Division of Allergy-Immunology, Johns Hopkins University, 7939 Honeygo Boulevard #219, Baltimore, MD 21236, USA
E-mail address: dgolden1@jhmi.edu

Immunol Allergy Clin N Am 35 (2015) 287–302
http://dx.doi.org/10.1016/j.iac.2015.01.007
0889-8561/15/$ – see front matter
immunology.theclinics.com

Systemic (generalized) reactions may cause any one or more of the signs and symptoms of anaphylaxis. Although the definition of anaphylaxis seems to exclude reactions involving only cutaneous systemic manifestations (urticaria, angioedema, pruritus, flush), these are included in this article because they must be considered in diagnosis and treatment of insect allergy as potential precursors of more severe anaphylactic reactions. There are also reports of chronic urticaria and cold urticaria developing after insect stings, usually without any immediate hypersensitivity reaction, and with uncertain risk of anaphylaxis to a future sting.[2,3] Unusual patterns of reaction have also been reported, including nephropathy, central and peripheral neurologic syndromes, idiopathic thrombocytopenic purpura, and rhabdomyolysis, but these are not IgE related.[4]

Systemic (generalized) allergic sting reactions result in cutaneous, vascular, or respiratory symptoms and signs, either singly or in any combination, with possible involvement of other less common target tissues. Cardiac anaphylaxis can also cause bradycardia, arrhythmias, angina, or myocardial infarction.[5] Hypotension or cardiac anaphylaxis without cutaneous signs or symptoms can easily be misdiagnosed.[6] Abdominal cramps are common, resulting from gastrointestinal tract or uterine smooth muscle contraction. There may be a greater chance of systemic reaction if there are multiple stings at one time, or if there are repeated stings in the same summer.[7] The onset of reactions is generally within 10 to 30 minutes of the sting. Abrupt onset after a sting may be related to an underlying mast-cell disorder.[8] Onset of symptoms 1 to 4 hours after a sting has been reported in a small number of cases.[9] In contrast with food anaphylaxis, the slower the onset of the sting reaction, the less likely it is to be life threatening.[9,10]

Whether anaphylaxis differs clinically between children and adults is unclear for most causes, but is known for insect-sting allergy, both in the clinical history and the natural history. Cutaneous symptoms are most common overall, affecting 80% of patients with systemic reactions to stings, in both adults and children; they are the sole manifestation in 15% of adults but in 60% of affected children.[11] Almost 50% of reactions in both children and adults included respiratory complaints. Symptoms and signs of hypotension were uncommon in children but occurred in more than 30% of adults, with half experiencing loss of consciousness (which is rare in children).[9,12] The clinical presentation can be vague and uncertain both during the reaction and in the history. To aid proper diagnosis and treatment, objective documentation should be made whenever possible, including description of cutaneous findings, vital signs, pulse oximetry, and air flow measurements.

Differential Diagnosis

Although a history of insect-sting anaphylaxis might be expected to be obvious, this is not always the case. When reactions have not been observed and treated by a physician, there can be uncertainty as to the true nature of the symptoms. Objective urticaria or angioedema (distant from the site of the sting), or documented hypotension, can confirm the diagnosis of anaphylaxis. The absence of cutaneous symptoms or signs, which occurs in 15% to 30% of cases of insect-sting anaphylaxis (more in adults than in children), does not rule out anaphylaxis, and has been associated with a higher frequency of hypotension and mastocytosis (particularly in male patients).[13] Non–IgE-mediated reactions can occur in patients with mastocytosis.

Subjective symptoms can occur that are convincing (eg, throat or chest discomfort, dyspnea, light-headedness) and must be assumed to be allergic when gleaned from the patient history. However, such reactions have often occurred under monitored sting challenge conditions when no objective abnormalities were found (ie, normal physical examination, vital signs, pulse oximetry, air flow measurement, and serum tryptase), making it unclear whether they are caused by allergic mast-cell mediator release.[14] Many of these symptoms are consistent with anxiety, but can also be related to hyperventilation or vocal cord dysfunction.

ETIOLOGY/PATHOPHYSIOLOGY

Stinging insects of the order Hymenoptera are the main cause of insect-related anaphylaxis. There are 3 families of Hymenoptera with clinical importance: the bees (honeybees, bumblebees), vespids (yellow jackets, hornets, wasps), and stinging ants (genus *Solenopsis* and others). Exposure to these insects is affected by geographic, environmental, and ecological factors. The Africanized honeybee (the so-called killer bee) is an aggressive hybrid resulting from an experiment intended to enhance honey production. The danger from the Africanized honeybees stems from the numbers of stings because of their swarm-and-attack behavior; their venom is no different from that of other honeybees. Imported fire ants arrived 75 years ago in Mobile, Alabama, and have rapidly become an increasing public health hazard in the south and southeast parts of the United States.[15,16] There have been increasing reports of anaphylaxis caused by other species of stinging ants in Asia and Australia.[17]

The immunochemical characteristics and immunogenetic relationships of the Hymenoptera venoms have been thoroughly studied.[18,19] Venoms contain multiple protein allergens, most having enzymatic activity. Honeybee venom is immunochemically distinct from that of the other Hymenoptera, but cross reactivity is often observed in serum IgE tests for honeybee and yellow jacket venoms because of the presence of cross reacting carbohydrate determinants (CCDs) on the native allergens.[20] Vespid venoms have a high degree of cross reactivity with each other and contain essentially the same allergens. Patients who are allergic to yellow jacket stings also have positive tests for hornet venom IgE in 95% of cases. *Polistes* wasps are not as closely related to the other vespids, and only 50% of patients allergic to yellow jackets or hornets have positive tests to wasp venom. Fire ant venoms are different in that they contain very little protein, in a suspension of alkaloid toxins that causes the characteristic vesicular eruption. The proteins in fire ant venoms are antigenically unique except for 1 that shows limited cross reactivity with a vespid allergen. The diagnostic and therapeutic materials currently supplied by commercial laboratories are fire ant whole-body extracts that, unlike the other insect whole-body extracts, show reasonable allergenic activity for diagnostic skin testing and for preventative immunotherapy.[21–23] The other 5 Hymenoptera products (honeybee, yellow jacket, yellow hornet, white-faced hornet, and *Polistes* wasp) are supplied as lyophilized venom protein extracts to be reconstituted using an albumin-saline diluent.

EPIDEMIOLOGY/NATURAL HISTORY

Knowledge of the epidemiology and natural history of Hymenoptera venom sensitivity is crucial in clinical decision making. Insect-sting allergy can occur at any age, often following several uneventful stings. Systemic allergic reactions are reported by up to 3% of adults, and almost 1% of children have a medical history of allergic sting reactions.[24,25] The frequency of large local reactions is uncertain, but is estimated at 10% in adults.[24,25] At least 40 fatal sting reactions occur each year in the United States.[10,26] Half of all fatal reactions occur with no history of previous sting reactions.[27] Many sting fatalities may be unrecognized and attributed to other causes. In some cases of unexplained sudden death in the summer, postmortem blood samples show the presence of both venom-specific IgE antibodies and increased serum tryptase level, suggesting a possible fatal sting reaction as the cause of death.[27,28] However, the presence of IgE antibodies to Hymenoptera venom is common. Sensitization to Hymenoptera venoms is common, but systemic sting reactions are much less common.[29] More than 30% of adults stung in the previous 3 months showed venom-specific IgE by skin test or serum test, and more than 20% of a random sample of adults tested positive to yellow jacket or honeybee venom, even though most had no history of allergic sting reactions, and almost all had been stung in the past.[25] Venom sensitivity in asymptomatic adults is often transient, disappearing more rapidly than it does in patients with a history of anaphylaxis. Of the subjects with initial positive skin tests, 30% to 60% became negative after 3 to 6 years. Those who remained positive showed a 17% frequency of a systemic reaction to a sting.[30]

Systemic reactions become progressively more severe with each sting in some cases, but this seems to be the exception rather than the rule. In children, a prospective long-term study showed that those with cutaneous systemic reactions had about a 10% chance of a similar or milder reaction, but only a 1% to 3% chance of a more severe reaction.[31] The findings were similar in a follow-up survey of the same pediatric cohort for 15 to 20 years.[32] In that study, children with moderate or severe anaphylaxis to stings who did not receive venom immunotherapy (VIT) still had a 32% frequency of anaphylaxis to recent stings.

In adults who have had previous systemic reactions to stings, a repeat sting causes another systemic reaction in 30% to 65% of cases, depending mainly on the severity of previous reactions, the level of venom sensitivity, and the species of insect.[14] Systemic reactions are more common with honeybee than vespid stings, more with hornets than yellow jackets, and more with some yellow jacket species (*Vespula maculifrons*) than with others (*Vespula germanica*). However, it has been noted that a patient can react to one sting and not another even from the same species. This difference may be caused by a 10-fold variability in the amount of venom injected by a vespid sting,[33] which can lead to a misleading impression that the patient is no longer allergic, only to have them react to a later sting.

In adults with a history of mild systemic reactions to stings, there has been less of a consensus on the risk of more severe reactions to future stings. In prospective sting challenge studies, less than 1% of the patients had reactions more severe than their past reactions.[14,34] In 2 retrospective surveys, there were a larger number of subjects who described worsening of the reaction with subsequent stings.[9,35] Allergic reactions to stings usually follow a predictable and individual pattern in each patient with severity being variable. Anaphylactic reactions to stings can occur even decades apart, with or without intervening stings.

Table 1 shows the risk of systemic reaction in untreated patients with a history of sting anaphylaxis and positive venom skin tests.

DIAGNOSIS
History

The history is paramount in diagnosis and must be elicited with insight and attention to detail. Patients usually fail to admit sting reactions without specific inquiry, often do not seek medical attention, and typically believe the reaction was a chance occurrence that could not happen again (because they have had many previous stings without reaction).[25] The history should include all previous stings, the time course of the reactions, and all associated symptoms and treatments. The reaction to any sting can be variable in occurrence and severity, even in individuals allergic to stings. Even without intervening stings, sensitization can persist for decades and result in subsequent

Table 1
Risk of systemic reaction in untreated patients with history of sting anaphylaxis and positive venom skin tests

Original Sting Reaction		Risk of Systemic Reaction (%)	
Severity	Age	1–9 y	10–20 y
No reaction	Adult	17	—
Large local	All	10	10
Cutaneous	Child	10	5
systemic	Adult	20	10
Anaphylaxis	Child	40	30
	Adult	60	40

From Golden DB. Insect Allergy. In: Adkinson NF Jr, Bochner BS, Burks AW, et al, editors. Middleton's allergy: principles and practice. 8th edition. Philadelphia: Elsevier; 2014:1266; with permission.

anaphylactic reactions to stings. If intervening stings have occurred without systemic reaction there could be less risk of subsequent severe reaction, but the species of insect is never certain to be the same as the underlying allergy, and the possibility of future anaphylaxis cannot be excluded when diagnostic tests reveal venom-specific IgE antibodies.[14]

The significance of the sting reaction can be overestimated or underestimated. Symptoms are sometimes exaggerated by fear, panic, exercise, heat, alcohol, or underlying cardiorespiratory disease. For this reason, objective documentation of the physical findings during the reaction should be sought (measurements of blood pressure or reduced air flow, observed urticaria). The history is sometimes of a sting reaction that occurred many years earlier and is poorly remembered. Even when the reaction was not severe, people have often been told by physicians that the next one will kill them.

Diagnostic Tests

Diagnostic tests are indicated in patients who have had systemic reactions to stings.[36] If the risk of future anaphylaxis is judged to be low (less than 10%) based on the history, diagnostic testing (and VIT) is not required; this is the case in patients with only large local reactions to stings, and in children who had only cutaneous systemic reactions. There are also patients who request venom testing because of fear of the reactions experienced by family members, friends, or others. Testing is not advised in such cases because of the frequent occurrence of positive venom tests in individuals who have previously been stung with no abnormal reaction.

However, skin tests are not a useful screening test and are not recommended in patients with no history of systemic allergic reaction to a sting. A screening test for insect allergy is desirable in order to prevent the morbidity and mortality of the initial anaphylactic episode; half of all fatal reactions occur without prior reactions to stings. Venom immunotherapy is indicated only in patients who have a history of a previous systemic reaction because venom skin tests are positive in many adults who have had previous stings and will have no reaction to a future sting.[29,30]

The preferred diagnostic method is venom skin testing because of its high degree of sensitivity and proven safety.[36,37] In vitro methods can be useful but are not as sensitive and can therefore yield false-negative results in more than 10% of cases. The standard method of skin testing is with the intradermal technique using the 5 Hymenoptera venom protein extracts (and/or whole-body extracts of imported fire ants). For Hymenoptera venom testing, intradermal tests are performed with venom concentrations in the range of 0.001 to 1.0 μg/mL to find the minimum concentration giving a positive result. Puncture tests at concentrations less than or equal to 100 μg/mL may be used initially for patients with a history of severe reactions to stings. Sensitization may have occurred to multiple venoms even when there has only been a reaction to a single insect; therefore, skin testing should be performed with a complete set of 5 Hymenoptera venoms, a negative diluent (HSA-saline) control, and a positive histamine control.

Skin test results are clearly positive in 65% to 85% of patients with a convincing history. Negative skin tests in history-positive patients can occur for several possible reasons. In the case of a remote sting reaction, this can be caused by loss of sensitivity. After a recent sting there could be a temporary refractory period of anergy for several weeks.[38] Venom skin tests also show unexplained variability over time such that tests can be negative on one occasion and positive on another.[39] It may be best to perform venom skin tests (or perform both skin tests and serum tests) on separate occasions before making the final therapeutic selection of venoms. Some cases of sting anaphylaxis seem to be non–IgE mediated and may be related to underlying mastocytosis or simply toxic mast-cell mediator release. Most important, the degree of skin test sensitivity does not correlate reliably with the degree of sting reaction.[14] The strongest skin tests often occur in patients who have had only large local reactions and have a low risk of anaphylaxis, whereas some patients who have had abrupt and near-fatal anaphylactic shock show only weak skin test (or specific serum IgE) sensitivity. About 25% of patients presenting for systemic allergic reactions to stings are skin test positive only at the 1.0-μg/mL concentration. Again, it is the history that is most predictive.

The detection of allergen-specific IgE antibodies in serum is less sensitive than skin testing, but is useful when skin tests cannot be done (patients with a severe skin condition or unavoidable medications that suppress skin tests). Another use of the serum IgE test is to resolve the discordance when skin tests are negative in patients with a history of a severe reaction to a sting. It is not clear whether there is any difference in prognostic value of skin tests and serum tests. Patients with negative skin tests and positive serum tests have been reported to have systemic reactions to subsequent stings, although the frequency may be lower than in patients with positive venom skin tests.[14]

Some investigators have suggested that sting challenge is the most specific diagnostic test, but others find this unethical and impractical.[34,40,41] Furthermore, a single negative challenge sting does not preclude anaphylaxis to a subsequent sting.[14,42] Newer approaches include either new materials (recombinant allergens) or new techniques (basophil activation tests). Recombinant venom allergens have been studied for serum IgE measurement in patients with dual sensitization to honey bee and yellow jacket venoms, in whom the tests can distinguish whether the patient is primarily allergic to just 1 of the venoms, or is allergic to both.[43–45] The recombinant venom allergens are free of the CCDs on the native venoms that may cause the serologic cross reactivity. Serum IgE tests with recombinant venom allergens do not show improved sensitivity, and have lower diagnostic accuracy than tests with the native venom extracts.[37] When multiple recombinant allergens are combined to approximate the repertoire of allergens in the native venom, the diagnostic sensitivity is improved but still not as good that of as the whole venom.

Basophil activation tests have been under development for many years. As a marker of susceptibility to basophil mediator release, these tests may provide clinically significant evidence of reactivity with, or potentially even without, specific IgE. The expression of basophil activation markers, particularly CD63, on exposure to very low concentrations of allergen has been reported to detect venom allergy in patients with no detectable venom-specific IgE on serum or skin tests, to predict efficacy of VIT, and to predict relapse after stopping VIT.[46–48] The methodology for performing and interpreting these tests has not yet been standardized, but it seems likely that they will become part of the diagnostic arsenal in the future.

Table 2 summarizes the diagnostic evaluation of insect-sting allergy.

RISK FACTORS FOR STING ANAPHYLAXIS

There are 2 elements of risk in insect-sting allergy: frequency and severity. The chance of a systemic reaction to stings is related to the frequency of exposure, the level of sensitivity on serum or skin tests for venom IgE, and the severity of previous reactions to stings **(Table 3)**.[14] The severity of sting anaphylaxis is not predicted reliably by the level of venom sensitivity on serum or skin tests but may be correlated with markers of basophil and mast-cell responses, such as the level of baseline serum tryptase.[49] The Spanish Mastocytosis Network has described a Red Española de Mastocitosis (REMA) score that predicts underlying mastocytosis in patients with insect-sting anaphylaxis who are male and have hypotensive shock reactions to stings without cutaneous manifestations.[13] Insect stings are the most common cause of anaphylaxis in patients with indolent systemic mastocytosis.[50] Baseline serum tryptase level is increased in 25% of patients with a history of hypotension after a sting, and in about 5% of patients with other systemic reactions to stings.[51] Mastocytosis and/or increased baseline tryptase level are associated with not only increased risk of severe reactions to stings but also increased risk of systemic reactions to VIT injections, increased risk of treatment failure, and increased risk of relapse after a VIT (including fatal anaphylaxis).[49,52–56] There is also early evidence that a low level of platelet-activating factor acetylhydrolase is correlated with severe and fatal anaphylaxis to foods or insect stings.[57,58]

Antihypertensive medications, particularly β-blockers, have been reported to increase the risk of a severe allergic reaction to a sting.[49] In the case of β-blockers, the concern is mainly the potential for epinephrine resistance requiring additional

Table 2
Diagnostic evaluation of insect-sting allergy

Purpose	History	Skin Test	Specific IgE	BAT	Recombinant Allergen	RAST-Inhibition	Tryptase Baseline
Diagnosis							
No reaction	X						
LLR	X						
Mild systemic reaction	X	X	X				
Anaphylaxis	X	X	X	X	X	X	X
Predict severe reaction (to stings or VIT)	X			X			X
Cross-reactivity (honeybee/ yellow jacket)					X	X	
Discontinue VIT	X			X			X

Abbreviations: BAT, basophil activation test; LLR, large local reaction; RAST, radio-allergosorbent test.

From Golden DB. Advances in diagnosis and management of insect sting allergy. Ann Allergy Asthma Immunol 2013;111:85; with permission.

Table 3
Predictors of risk of systemic reaction to insect stings

Natural History	Markers
Severity of previous reaction	Venom skin test
Insect species	Venom-specific IgE
Age/Gender	Basophil activation test
No urticaria/angioedema	Baseline serum tryptase value
Medications	PAF acetylhydrolase
Multiple or sequential stings	Angiotensin-converting enzyme

Abbreviation: PAF, platelet-activating factor.
From Golden DB. Insect Allergy. In: Adkinson NF Jr, Bochner BS, Burks AW, et al, editors. Middleton's allergy: principles and practice. 8th edition. Philadelphia: Elsevier; 2014:1266; with permission.

epinephrine and intravenous (IV) fluids. If the patient remains unresponsive to epinephrine this may be overcome with glucagon injection. Angiotensin-converting enzyme inhibitors may increase the risk of angioedema with airway obstruction. Despite the convincing evidence to support these concerns in some studies, there are other reports that find no correlations.[8] There has also been concern that stopping β-blocker medication may create a greater risk than continuing the medication during VIT.[6]

ACUTE TREATMENT

Treatment of insect-sting anaphylaxis is no different from treating other causes of anaphylaxis, requiring immediate epinephrine injection and potentially IV fluids and oxygen.[36,59] In the presence of hypotensive symptoms, recumbent posture is of critical importance.[60] Biphasic and protracted anaphylaxis have been reported with insect stings, so medical observation should extend for 3 to 6 hours depending on severity. Some individuals are resistant to epinephrine, especially those on β-blocker medication. Nevertheless, the risk of stopping β-blockers in patients with cardiac disease may exceed the risk of continuing the drugs.[6] Patients discharged from emergency care after anaphylaxis should receive instruction about the appropriate use of an epinephrine autoinjector, and recommendations for an allergy consultation and preventative treatment. Patients should be specifically informed that VIT is routinely available and gives rapid protection and ultimately a cure (tolerance) in most cases. Patients should understand that using the epinephrine is not a substitute for emergency medical attention (in case of persistent or recurrent anaphylaxis), that the epinephrine is not dangerous at the recommended dose, and that delay in the use of epinephrine can increase the risk of fatal anaphylaxis.[61]

PREVENTION
Precautions

Individuals susceptible to allergic reactions to stings should avoid related exposures, particularly outdoor foods and drinks that attract or harbor stinging insects. However, excessive fear impairs quality of life and can be considered among the indications for VIT in patients who are otherwise at low risk for anaphylaxis.[62,63] When to carry or use an epinephrine injector depends on the clinical setting. Although having an emergency injector is reassuring to some individuals, it is frightening to others and conveys a concern about possible dangerous reactions to stings. Many experts suggest that an injector is not necessary when the chance of a systemic reaction is only 5% to 10%, such as in large local reactors, children with cutaneous systemic reactions, and patients who are receiving or have completed VIT. In contrast, some clinicians think that even a 1% chance of anaphylaxis warrants carrying epinephrine, even if it does not warrant VIT. Having an epinephrine injector does not improve the quality of life, whereas VIT does. This distinction has been shown not only in patients with moderate to severe sting anaphylaxis but even in those with cutaneous reactions.[64] Most insect allergic patients can be advised to keep an epinephrine injector at the ready when stung, but may not need to use it if the reaction does not occur or remains limited to mild (cutaneous) symptoms. Some patients have had rapid onset of severe reactions and (until immunized) should potentially use epinephrine immediately after being stung.

Venom Immunotherapy

One of the only types of anaphylaxis for which immunotherapy has been proved to be highly effective is insect-sting allergy. VIT has been the most useful model for the elucidation of the mechanisms of allergen immunotherapy. VIT has also proved to be the most highly effective form of immunotherapy at inducing full and reliable clinical protection and, ultimately, a lasting tolerance.

The indications for VIT require a history of previous systemic allergic reaction to a sting and a positive diagnostic test for venom-specific IgE. Such individuals have a 30% to 65% chance of systemic reaction to a subsequent sting.[34,65,66] This range is related to several factors as described earlier. Children do not always outgrow insect allergy, and those with moderate or severe systemic reactions should receive VIT. One study found that without VIT such children still have up to 30% chance of reaction to a sting even decades later.[32]

A low risk (<10%) has been reported in children and adults with a history of large local reactions, and in children with systemic reactions limited to cutaneous signs and symptoms (with no respiratory or circulatory manifestations).[1,31,32,67] Venom immunotherapy is not required in these low-risk cases, but some patients still request treatment because of their fear of reaction and the impact on their quality of life. Adults with cutaneous systemic reactions also seem to have a low risk of progression to anaphylaxis, but there are conflicting reports suggesting that the risk might justify the recommendation of VIT in such patients. However, there is no test that predicts which patients will progress to more severe reactions. Even intervening stings without reaction do not necessarily ensure that there will be no reaction to a later sting.

Initial VIT can follow any of several recommended schedules. The common modified-rush regimen is more rapid than traditional regimens, achieving the 100-µg maintenance dose with 8 weekly injections, instead of taking 4 to 6 months. With these regimens, adverse reactions are no more common than in traditional regimens of inhalant allergen immunotherapy, and both regimens are equally effective. Even rush regimens of 2 to 3 days are not associated with a higher frequency of adverse reactions to venom injections.[68–70] Ultrarush VIT is clearly associated with increased risk of anaphylactic adverse effects.[71]

Treatment is usually recommended with each of the venoms giving a positive skin test. Therapy is 98% effective in preventing systemic allergic reactions to stings when treatment includes mixed vespid venoms (300-µg total dose), but complete protection is achieved in only 75% to 90% of patients using 100 µg of any single venom (eg, honeybee, yellow jacket, or *Polistes* wasp). Fire ant immunotherapy using whole-body extracts has been reported to be reasonably safe and effective, and should be used in cases of significant systemic reaction, although there have been no controlled trials.[22,23] Fire ant venoms are not available for diagnosis or treatment, but jack jumper ant VIT was very successful in a controlled clinical trial in Australia.[72]

Adverse reactions to VIT occur no more frequently than with inhalant allergen immunotherapy.[73,74] Systemic symptoms occur in 10% to 15% of patients during the initial weeks of treatment with semirush or traditional regimens. Most reactions are mild, and fewer than half require epinephrine injection. Virtually all patients can achieve the full dose even after initial systemic reactions. In the unusual case of repeated systemic reactions to injections even after adjustment of the dose schedule, VIT up to maintenance doses has been achieved using inpatient rush VIT, and in some cases with omalizumab pretreatment. Large local reactions to injections are common, occurring in up to 50% of patients. Unlike standard inhalant immunotherapy, the uniform target dose in VIT may make it necessary to advance the dose if there are large local reactions, beyond what might otherwise be considered the maximum tolerated dose. Large local reactions can be reduced by pretreatment with antihistamines and leukotriene modifiers without affecting efficacy.[75,76] Efficacy may be improved by pretreatment with antihistamines.[75]

Venom immunotherapy has been the most productive model for investigation of the mechanisms of immunotherapy. Venom IgE levels increase initially with treatment, then decline steadily over time toward very low levels after 5 to 10 years. Venom immunoglobulin G (IgG) levels generally increase with treatment, and have been correlated with clinical protection.[77,78] The IgG response is a downstream marker of interleukin-10 production, which in turn reflects changes in regulatory T-cell populations and dendritic cells.[79,80] However, the determinants and markers of long-term immune tolerance after immunotherapy remain elusive.

Maintenance doses of VIT are administered every 4 weeks for at least a year. Most experts agree that the maintenance interval then may be increased to every 6 weeks for at least a year, and later to every 8 weeks.[36] Venom skin tests or serum IgE tests are repeated periodically, usually every 2 to 3 years, to determine when there has been a significant decline in sensitivity. Skin tests generally remain unchanged in the first 2 to 3 years, but show a significant decline after 4 to 6 years. Less than 20% of patients are skin test negative after 5 years, but 50% to 60% become negative after 7 to 10 years (although most remain positive on serum IgE tests).[81,82] Patients who continue VIT beyond 4 to 5 years can be safely and effectively treated every 12 weeks.[83]

The duration of VIT is indefinite according to the recommendation in the product package insert. Initial efforts to stop treatment when the serum IgE became negative were successful, but only a few patients become IgE-negative within 5 years of treatment.[84,85] However extended study of a large number of adults has shown that when VIT is stopped after 5 years, the chance of a systemic reaction remains 10% for each sting even more than 10 years after stopping treatment, and even if skin tests become negative.[82,86] When sting reactions occur after stopping VIT, most are mild and almost always less severe than the pretreatment reaction. A higher frequency of relapse occurs in patients who had very severe (near-fatal) sting reactions before therapy, those who had a systemic reaction during therapy (to a sting or a venom injection), those with honeybee allergy, those with increased baseline serum tryptase level, and those who had less than 5 years of therapy.[82,87–89] Patients with any of these high-risk characteristics may need to be treated indefinitely, but there are no data on the outcome in these patients after more than 15 years of treatment. Some patients prefer to continue venom treatment for security and improved quality of life, especially those with frequent, unavoidable, or occupational exposure. Children who have had 3 to 5 years of VIT have a very low chance of systemic reaction even 10 to 20 years after stopping treatment.[32]

CURRENT CONTROVERSIES/FUTURE CONSIDERATIONS

There remain a few areas of controversy and ongoing investigation in insect-sting allergy. There is a need for new and better diagnostic and prognostic tests that can distinguish those individuals who will have severe reactions to future stings from those who have minimal risk despite similar levels of venom IgE. Such a test might also serve as a screening test that could prevent anaphylaxis to future stings, including the fatalities that occur on the first reaction that are currently not preventable. There is also a need for a test that could distinguish patients who have achieved permanent tolerance after years of VIT from those whose protection will wane if they stop treatment.

There is a need to clarify the relative risk of more severe reactions in adults who have had only mild systemic reactions to stings. At present, these patients are advised that it would be prudent to undergo VIT, although outside the United States this is not the case.

SUMMARY

Anaphylaxis to insect stings has occurred in 3% of adults and can be fatal even on the first reaction. Large local reactions are more frequent but rarely dangerous. The chance of a systemic reaction to a sting is low (5%–10%) in those with large local reactions and in children with mild (cutaneous) systemic reactions, and varies between 30% and 65% in adults with systemic reactions depending on the severity of previous sting reactions. Venom skin tests are most accurate for diagnosis but measurement of serum-specific IgE is an important complementary test. The level of venom IgE detected by the skin test or serum test does not reliably predict the severity of a sting reaction. Venom sensitization can be detected in 25% of adults, so the history is most important in clinical evaluation. Venom immunotherapy is 75% to 98% effective in preventing sting anaphylaxis. Most patients can discontinue treatment after 5 years, with very low residual risk of a severe sting reaction.

Anaphylaxis to insect stings is unique in some ways, especially its mode of antigen exposure, its well-described natural history, its milder relatives (large local and cutaneous reactions), and its remarkable response to immunotherapy. Familiarity with these features permits better recognition and prevention of insect-sting anaphylaxis. There is a need to educate the public and health care professionals about the availability, efficacy, and safety of VIT.

There is a need for improved accuracy in diagnostic tests for insect-sting allergy, which may be achieved with dialyzed venoms, recombinant venoms allergens, basophil activation tests, or other in vitro procedures. There remains a need to determine the best predictive factors that distinguish patients who would react to stings from those who are sensitized but do not have anaphylaxis. Such a test would identify those individuals who are at risk before their first reaction occurs, those who are immunized but have incomplete protection, and those who will have increased risk of reaction if they discontinue VIT. Clinicians could then target the therapy to those most likely to benefit and spare patients who are sensitized but are not in danger. Such insight may come from studying large local reactors (who are highly sensitized but have the lowest risk of anaphylaxis), untreated patients who do not react to a challenge sting, and patients who relapse after stopping VIT.

REFERENCES

1. Graft DF, Schuberth KC, Kagey-Sobotka A, et al. A Prospective study of the natural history of large local reactions following Hymenoptera stings in children. J Pediatr 1984;104:664–8.

2. Hogendijk S, Hauser C. Wasp sting-associated cold urticaria. Allergy 1997;52: 1145–6.
3. Wong CC, Borici-Mazi R. Delayed-onset cold anaphylaxis after Hymenoptera sting. Ann Allergy Asthma Immunol 2012;109:77–8.
4. Reisman RE. Unusual reactions to insect stings. Curr Opin Allergy Clin Immunol 2005;5:355–8.
5. Triggiani M, Patella V, Staiano RI, et al. Allergy and the cardiovascular system. Clin Exp Immunol 2008;153(Suppl 1):7–11.
6. Muller UR. Cardiovascular disease and anaphylaxis. Curr Opin Allergy Clin Immunol 2007;7:337–41.
7. Pucci S, Antonicelli L, Bilo MB, et al. The short interval between two stings as a risk factor for developing Hymenoptera venom allergy. Allergy 1994;49:894–6.
8. Stoevesandt J, Hain J, Kerstan A, et al. Over- and underestimated parameters in severe Hymenoptera venom-induced anaphylaxis: cardiovascular medication and absence of urticaria/angioedema. J Allergy Clin Immunol 2012;130: 698–704.
9. Lockey RF, Turkeltaub PC, Baird-Warren IA, et al. The Hymenoptera venom study. I. 1979-1982: demographic and history-sting data. J Allergy Clin Immunol 1988; 82:370–81.
10. Barnard JH. Studies of 400 Hymenoptera sting deaths in the United States. J Allergy Clin Immunol 1973;52:259–64.
11. Schuberth KC, Lichtenstein LM, Kagey-Sobotka A, et al. An epidemiologic study of insect allergy in children. I. Characteristics of the disease. J Pediatr 1982;100: 546–51.
12. Insect Allergy Committee, American Academy of Allergy. Insect sting allergy, cooperative study. JAMA 1965;193:115–20.
13. Alvarez-Twose I, Gonzalez-de-Olano D, Sanchez-Munoz L, et al. Clinical, biological and molecular characteristics of systemic mast cell disorders presenting with severe mediator-related symptoms. J Allergy Clin Immunol 2010;125:1269–78.
14. Golden DB, Breisch NL, Hamilton RG, et al. Clinical and entomological factors influence the outcome of sting challenge studies. J Allergy Clin Immunol 2006; 117:670–5.
15. Kemp SF, deShazo RD, Moffitt JE, et al. Expanding habitat of the imported fire ant: a public health concern. J Allergy Clin Immunol 2000;105:683–91.
16. Tracy JM, Demain JG, Quinn JM, et al. The natural history of exposure to the imported fire ant. J Allergy Clin Immunol 1995;95:824–8.
17. Shek LP, Ngiam NS, Lee BW. Ant allergy in Asia and Australia. Curr Opin Allergy Clin Immunol 2004;4:325–8.
18. Hoffman DR. Hymenoptera venoms: composition, standardization, stability. In: Levine MI, Lockey RF, editors. Monograph on insect allergy. 4th edition. Milwaukee (WI): American Academy of Allergy Asthma and Immunology; 2004. p. 37–53.
19. King TP, Spangfort MD. Structure and biology of stinging insect venom allergens. Int Arch Allergy Immunol 2000;123:99–106.
20. Hemmer W, Frocke M, Kolarich K, et al. Antibody binding to venom carbohydrates is a frequent cause for double positivity to honeybee and yellow jacket venom in patients with stinging insect allergy. J Allergy Clin Immunol 2001;108: 1045–52.
21. Hoffman DR, Jacobson RS, Schmidt M, et al. Allergens in Hymenoptera venoms. XXIII. Venom content of imported fire ant whole body extracts. Ann Allergy 1991; 66:29–31.

22. Freeman TM, Hyghlander R, Ortiz A, et al. Imported fire ant immunotherapy: effectiveness of whole body extracts. J Allergy Clin Immunol 1992;90:210–5.
23. Steigelman DA, Freeman TM. Imported fire ant allergy: case presentation and review of incidence, prevalence, diagnosis and current treatment. Ann Allergy Asthma Immunol 2013;111:242–5.
24. Bilo BM, Bonifazi F. Epidemiology of insect-venom anaphylaxis. Curr Opin Allergy Clin Immunol 2008;8:330–7.
25. Golden DB, Marsh DG, Kagey-Sobotka A, et al. Epidemiology of insect venom sensitivity. JAMA 1989;262:240–4.
26. Graft DF. Insect sting allergy. Med Clin North Am 2006;90:211–32.
27. Hoffman DR. Fatal reactions to Hymenoptera stings. Allergy Asthma Proc 2003; 24:123–7.
28. Schwartz HJ, Sutheimer C, Gauerke B, et al. Venom-specific IgE antibodies in postmortem sera from victims of sudden unexpected death [abstract]. J Allergy Clin Immunol 1984;73:189.
29. Sturm GJ, Kranzelbinder B, Schuster C, et al. Sensitization to Hymenoptera venoms is common, but systemic sting reactions are rare. J Allergy Clin Immunol 2014;133:1635–43.e1.
30. Golden DB, Marsh DG, Freidhoff LR, et al. Natural history of Hymenoptera venom sensitivity in adults. J Allergy Clin Immunol 1997;100:760–6.
31. Valentine MD, Schuberth KC, Kagey-Sobotka A, et al. The value of immunotherapy with venom in children with allergy to insect stings. N Engl J Med 1990;323:1601–3.
32. Golden DB, Kagey-Sobotka A, Norman PS, et al. Outcomes of allergy to insect stings in children with and without venom immunotherapy. N Engl J Med 2004; 351:668–74.
33. Hoffman DR, Jacobson RS. Allergens in Hymenoptera venom. XII. How much protein is in a sting? Ann Allergy 1984;52:276–8.
34. vanderLinden PG, Hack CE, Struyvenberg A, et al. Insect-sting challenge in 324 subjects with a previous anaphylactic reaction: current criteria for insect-venom hypersensitivity do not predict the occurrence and the severity of anaphylaxis. J Allergy Clin Immunol 1994;94:151–9.
35. Golden DB, Langlois J, Valentine MD. Treatment failures with whole body extract therapy of insect sting allergy. JAMA 1981;246:2460–3.
36. Golden DB, Moffitt J, Nicklas RA, American Academy of Allergy, Asthma & Immunology (AAAAI). Stinging insect hypersensitivity: a practice parameter update 2011. J Allergy Clin Immunol 2011;127:852–4.
37. Golden DB. Advances in diagnosis and management of insect sting allergy. Ann Allergy Asthma Immunol 2013;111:84–9.
38. Goldberg A, Confino-Cohen R. Timing of venom skin tests and IgE determinations after insect sting anaphylaxis. J Allergy Clin Immunol 1997;100: 183–4.
39. Graif Y, Confino-Cohen R, Goldberg A. Reproducibility of skin testing and serum venom-specific IgE in Hymenoptera venom allergy. Ann Allergy 2006;96:24–9.
40. Reisman RE. Intentional diagnostic insect sting challenges: a medical and ethical issue [letter]. J Allergy Clin Immunol 1993;91:1100.
41. Rueff F, Przybilla B, Muller U, et al. The sting challenge test in Hymenoptera venom allergy. Allergy 1996;51:216–25.
42. Franken HH, Dubois AE, Minkema HJ, et al. Lack of reproducibility of a single negative sting challenge response in the assessment of anaphylactic risk in patients with suspected yellow jacket hypersensitivity. J Allergy Clin Immunol 1994;93:431–6.

43. Eberlein B, Krischan L, Darsow U, et al. Double positivity to bee and wasp venom: improved diagnostic procedure by recombinant allergen-based IgE testing and basophil activation test including data about cross-reactive carbohydrate determinants. J Allergy Clin Immunol 2012;130:155–61.
44. Muller UR, Johansen N, Petersen AB, et al. Hymenoptera venom allergy: analysis of double positivity to honey bee and Vespula venom by estimation of IgE antibodies to species-specific major allergens Api m1 and Ves v5. Allergy 2009; 64:543–8.
45. Muller UR, Schmid-Grendelmeier P, Hausmann O, et al. IgE to recombinant allergens Api m 1, Ves v 1, and Ves v 5 distinguish double sensitization from cross-reaction in venom allergy. Allergy 2012;67:1069–73.
46. Eberlein-Konig B, Schmidt-Leidescher C, Behrendt H, et al. Predicting side-effects in venom immunotherapy by basophil activation? Allergy 2006;61:897.
47. Kucera P, Cvackova M, Hulikova K, et al. Basophil activation can predict clinical sensitivity in patients after venom immunotherapy. J Investig Allergol Clin Immunol 2010;20:110–6.
48. Zitnik SE, Vesel T, Avcin T, et al. Monitoring honeybee venom immunotherapy in children with the basophil activation test. Pediatr Allergy Immunol 2012;23: 166–72.
49. Rueff F, Przybilla B, Bilo MB, et al. Predictors of severe systemic anaphylactic reactions in patients with Hymenoptera venom allergy: importance of baseline serum tryptase - a study of the EAACI Interest Group on Insect Venom Hypersensitivity. J Allergy Clin Immunol 2009;124:1047–54.
50. Niedoszytko M, deMonchy J, vanDoormaal JJ, et al. Mastocytosis and insect venom allergy: diagnosis, safety and efficacy of venom immunotherapy. Allergy 2009;64:1237–45.
51. Bonadonna P, Perbellini O, Passalacqua G, et al. Clonal mast cell disorders in patients with systemic reactions to Hymenoptera stings and increased serum tryptase levels. J Allergy Clin Immunol 2009;123:680–6.
52. Haeberli G, Bronnimann M, Hunziker T, et al. Elevated basal serum tryptase and hymenoptera venom allergy: relation to severity of sting reactions and to safety and efficacy of venom immunotherapy. Clin Exp Allergy 2003;33:1216–20.
53. Kucharewicz I, Bodzenta-Lukaszyk A, Szymanski W, et al. Basal serum tryptase level correlates with severity of Hymenoptera sting and age. J Investig Allergol Clin Immunol 2007;17:65–9.
54. Muller UR. Elevated baseline serum tryptase, mastocytosis and anaphylaxis. Clin Exp Allergy 2009;39:620–2.
55. Rueff F, Przybilla B, Bilo MB, et al. Predictors of side effects during the buildup phase of venom immunotherapy for Hymenoptera venom allergy: the importance of baseline serum tryptase. J Allergy Clin Immunol 2010;126:105–11.
56. Oude-Elberink J, deMonchy J, Kors J, et al. Fatal anaphylaxis after a yellow jacket sting despite venom immunotherapy in two patients with mastocytosis. J Allergy Clin Immunol 1997;99:153–4.
57. Pravettoni V, Piantanida M, Primavesi L, et al. Basal platelet-activating factor acetylhydrolase: prognostic marker of severe Hymenoptera venom anaphylaxis. J Allergy Clin Immunol 2014;133:1218–20.
58. Vadas P, Gold M, Perelman B, et al. Platelet-activating factor, PAF acetylhydrolase, and severe anaphylaxis. N Engl J Med 2008;358:28–35.
59. Lieberman P, Nicklas RA, Oppenheimer J, et al. The diagnosis and management of anaphylaxis practice parameter: 2010 update. J Allergy Clin Immunol 2010; 126:477–80.

60. Pumphrey RS. Fatal posture in anaphylactic shock. J Allergy Clin Immunol 2003; 112:451–2.
61. Clark S, Long AA, Gaeta TJ, et al. Multicenter study of emergency department visits for insect sting allergies. J Allergy Clin Immunol 2005;116:643–9.
62. Oude-Elberink JN, deMonchy JG, vanderHeide S, et al. Venom immunotherapy improves health-related quality of life in yellow jacket allergic patients. J Allergy Clin Immunol 2002;110:174–82.
63. Oude-Elberink JN, vanderHeide S, Guyatt GH, et al. Analysis of the burden of treatment in patients receiving an Epi-Pen for yellow jacket anaphylaxis. J Allergy Clin Immunol 2006;118:699–704.
64. Oude-Elberink JN, vanderHeide S, Guyatt GH, et al. Immunotherapy improves health-related quality of life in adult patients with dermal reactions following yellow jacket stings. Clin Exp Allergy 2009;39:883–9.
65. Hunt KJ, Valentine MD, Sobotka AK, et al. A controlled trial of immunotherapy in insect hypersensitivity. N Engl J Med 1978;299:157–61.
66. Reisman RE. Natural history of insect sting allergy: relationship of severity of symptoms of initial sting anaphylaxis to re-sting reactions. J Allergy Clin Immunol 1992;90:335–9.
67. Mauriello PM, Barde SH, Georgitis JW, et al. Natural history of large local reactions from stinging insects. J Allergy Clin Immunol 1984;74:494–8.
68. Bernstein JA, Kagan SL, Bernstein DI, et al. Rapid venom immunotherapy is safe for routine use in the treatment of patients with Hymenoptera anaphylaxis. Ann Allergy 1994;73:423–8.
69. Birnbaum J, Charpin D, Vervloet D. Rapid Hymenoptera venom immunotherapy: comparative safety of three protocols. Clin Exp Allergy 1993;23:226–30.
70. Tankersley MS, Walker RL, Butler WK, et al. Safety and efficacy of an imported fire ant rush immunotherapy protocol with and without prophylactic treatment. J Allergy Clin Immunol 2002;109:556–62.
71. Brown SG, Wiese MD, vanEeden P, et al. Ultrarush versus semirush initiation of insect venom immunotherapy: a randomized controlled trial. J Allergy Clin Immunol 2012;130:162–8.
72. Brown SG, Wiese MD, Blackman KE, et al. Ant venom immunotherapy: a double-blind placebo-controlled crossover trial. Lancet 2003;361:1001–6.
73. Lockey RF, Turkeltaub PC, Olive ES, et al. The Hymenoptera venom study III: safety of venom immunotherapy. J Allergy Clin Immunol 1990;86:775–80.
74. Mosbech H, Muller U. Side effects of insect venom immunotherapy: results from an EAACI study. Allergy 2000;55:1005–10.
75. Muller UR, Jutel M, Reimers A, et al. Clinical and immunologic effects of H1 antihistamine preventive medication during honeybee venom immunotherapy. J Allergy Clin Immunol 2008;122:1001–7.
76. Wohrl S, Gamper S, Hemmer W, et al. Premedication with montelukast reduces large local reactions of allergen immunotherapy. Int Arch Allergy Immunol 2007;144:137–42.
77. Golden DB, Lawrence ID, Kagey-Sobotka A, et al. Clinical correlation of the venom-specific IgG antibody level during maintenance venom immunotherapy. J Allergy Clin Immunol 1992;90:386–93.
78. Varga EM, Francis JN, Zach MS, et al. Time course of serum inhibitory activity for facilitated allergen-IgE binding during bee venom immunotherapy in children. Clin Exp Allergy 2009;39:1353–7.
79. Dreschler K, Bratke K, Petermann S, et al. Impact of immunotherapy on blood dendritic cells in patients with Hymenoptera venom allergy. J Allergy Clin Immunol 2011;127:487–94.

80. Ozdemir C, Kucuksezer UC, Akdis M, et al. Mechanisms of immunotherapy to wasp and bee venom. Clin Exp Allergy 2011;41:1226–34.
81. Golden DB, Kwiterovich KA, Kagey-Sobotka A, et al. Discontinuing venom immunotherapy: outcome after five years. J Allergy Clin Immunol 1996;97:579–87.
82. Golden DB, Kwiterovich KA, Addison BA, et al. Discontinuing venom immunotherapy: extended observations. J Allergy Clin Immunol 1998;101:298–305.
83. Cavalucci E, Ramondo S, Renzetti A, et al. Maintenance venom immunotherapy administered at a 3 month interval preserves safety and efficacy and improves adherence. J Investig Allergol Clin Immunol 2010;20:63–8.
84. Muller U, Berchtold E, Helbling A. Honeybee venom allergy: results of a sting challenge 1 year after stopping venom immunotherapy in 86 patients. J Allergy Clin Immunol 1991;87:702–9.
85. Reisman RE, Lantner R. Further observations of stopping venom immunotherapy: comparison of patients stopped because of a fall in serum venom-specific IgE to insignificant levels with patients stopped prematurely by self-choice. J Allergy Clin Immunol 1989;83:1049–54.
86. Golden DB, Kagey-Sobotka A, Lichtenstein LM. Survey of patients after discontinuing venom immunotherapy. J Allergy Clin Immunol 2000;105:385–90.
87. Lerch E, Muller U. Long-term protection after stopping venom immunotherapy. J Allergy Clin Immunol 1998;101:606–12.
88. Muller U, Helbling A, Berchtold E. Immunotherapy with honeybee venom and yellow jacket venom is different regarding efficacy and safety. J Allergy Clin Immunol 1992;89:529–35.
89. Reisman RE. Duration of venom immunotherapy: relationship to the severity of symptoms of initial insect sting anaphylaxis. J Allergy Clin Immunol 1993;92:831–6.

Anaphylaxis to Drugs

 CrossMark

Merin Kuruvilla, MD[a], David A. Khan, MD[b],*

KEYWORDS

- Anaphylaxis • Drug • Penicillin • NSAID • Radiocontrast • Vocal cord dysfunction
- Proton pump inhibitor • Cephalosporin

KEY POINTS

- Drug-induced anaphylaxis is the most common cause of fatal anaphylaxis, with antibiotics and radiocontrast accounting for most fatalities.
- Vocal cord dysfunction can mimic anaphylaxis and is often overlooked as a cause leading to poor outcomes. Challenge with the culprit drug or drugs followed by laryngoscopy helps confirm the diagnosis.
- Nonsteroidal anti-inflammatory drug (NSAID) anaphylaxis is typically drug-specific, and other tolerated NSAIDs can be confirmed via graded challenge. Evidence for aspirin as a cause of anaphylaxis is lacking.
- Most patients with anaphylaxis from β-lactams can tolerate other classes of β-lactams. Skin testing and drug challenges can confirm tolerance to other β-lactam antibiotics.
- Immunoglobulin E (IgE)-mediated reactions may occur with nonionic radiocontrast media. Premedication regimens are not completely effective. The role of skin testing in the evaluation of patients with radiocontrast anaphylaxis is still evolving but should be considered.

INTRODUCTION

Anaphylaxis is a rapid-onset, multisystem hypersensitivity reaction with a potentially fatal outcome. It most often represents an immunologic (immunoglobulin E [IgE] or non-IgE-mediated) or nonimmunologic reaction to certain antigens, resulting in mast cell and basophil degranulation. In the context of medication allergies, it is mostly mediated by antigen-specific IgE responses, but other mechanisms have been well characterized, and the label of anaphylaxis encompasses all of these clinical syndromes.

The authors have nothing to disclose.
[a] Atlanta ENT, 5555 Peachtree Dunwoody Rd, Suite 125, Atlanta, GA-30342, USA; [b] Division of Allergy & Immunology, Department of Internal Medicine, University of Texas Southwestern Medical Center, 5323 Harry Hines Blvd, Dallas, TX 75390-8859, USA
* Corresponding author.
E-mail address: dave.khan@utsouthwestern.edu

Immunol Allergy Clin N Am 35 (2015) 303–319
http://dx.doi.org/10.1016/j.iac.2015.01.008   **immunology.theclinics.com**
0889-8561/15/$ – see front matter © 2015 Elsevier Inc. All rights reserved.

EPIDEMIOLOGY

The population prevalence, or incidence, of anaphylaxis has been difficult to quantify because of a lack of consensus on the definition of anaphylaxis, and analysis of different sample populations. Recent US studies have added important information on the epidemiology of drug-induced anaphylaxis.

Using a US nationwide cross-sectional telephone survey, the prevalence of anaphylaxis in the general adult population was 1.6% with medications being the most common trigger (35%).[1] Another US study using a pediatric emergency department (ED) database over a period of 5 years estimated that anaphylaxis is responsible for 0.18% of ED visits in the United States.[2] Excluding pediatric cohorts (wherein foods are the most common trigger), medications are the most frequent cause of fatal anaphylaxis in reports from the United States, as well as the United Kingdom, Australia, and New Zealand.[3]

In conjunction with an increasing worldwide incidence of anaphylaxis overall, drug-induced anaphylaxis admissions also increased by ~150% during the 8-year period studied in an Australian ED database.[4] In the same study, severe reactions (associated with hypotension) were more likely to be medication-induced ($P<.05$). This phenomenon is presumably in parallel with the increasing treatment of patients with multiple courses of sensitizing medications.

Medications are typically cited as among the most common triggers of fatal reactions. This finding was confirmed in a recent US study of fatal anaphylaxis (analyzed by coding of death certificates) by Jerschow and colleagues,[3] wherein 58.8% of fatal anaphylaxis were drug-induced. Unfortunately, the culprit drug was not specified in ~75% of these fatal drug-induced anaphylaxis cases. Among the ~25% of cases where a drug was identified, antibiotics accounted for 40% of the fatal episodes—most often penicillins, followed by cephalosporins, sulfa-containing drugs, and macrolides. Radiocontrast agents accounted for 27% of fatalities with antineoplastic drugs attributed to 12.5%. The remainder of culprit drugs was identified as serum, opiates, antihypertensives, nonsteroidal anti-inflammatory drugs (NSAIDs), and anesthetic agents.

RISK FACTORS

Clinical factors increasing the risk of drug-induced anaphylaxis are outlined in **Box 1**.

Demographic Factors

Of various demographic factors, older age has been associated with both higher rates of drug-induced anaphylaxis ($P<.001$)[3] and an increased risk of severe reactions.[5,6] African American race has also been associated with a higher prevalence of fatal drug-induced anaphylaxis.[3]

Banerji and colleagues[7] recently described the characteristics of 716 patients with drug-induced anaphylaxis in another ED database, most of whom were female (71%). In light of this conspicuous female predominance, it was postulated that female hormones may impact drug sensitization and the severity of associated allergic reactions. However, in the aforementioned study by Jerschow and colleagues,[3] there was no significant difference in rates of fatal drug-induced anaphylaxis between sexes.

Genetic Susceptibility

Decreased activity, or deficiency, of platelet-activating factor (PAF) acetylhydrolase, the enzyme that inactivates PAF, has been described as a risk factor for severe and

---

Box 1
Clinical factors increasing the risk of drug-induced anaphylaxis

- Demographics:
  - Female sex
  - Elderly age: increased risk of fatal reactions
  - African American race
- Genetics:
  - Reduced PAF-AH activity, leading to elevated PAF levels
- Comorbidities:
  - Mastocytosis and other mast cell disorders
- Concurrent medications:
  - β-Adrenergic blocking agents
  - ACE-Is
  - ARB
  - Monoamine oxidase inhibitors
  - PPIs

---

fatal anaphylaxis in foods.[8] Recently, decreased PAF acetylhydrolase has been reported with drug-induced anaphylaxis, including oral medication anaphylaxis.[6]

Clinical Comorbidities

The role of atopy in predisposing to drug-induced anaphylaxis is controversial. In general, although atopic diseases are a risk factor for anaphylaxis triggered by food, exercise, and latex, they are not considered to increase the risk of drug-induced episodes. However, oft-cited literature from Northern Europe from the 1960s reported an association with "allergy" and deaths from penicillin. On closer inspection of this literature, the determination of "allergy" and interpretation of the data are questionable. Bertelsen and Dalgaard[9] reported on 20 cases of fatal penicillin anaphylaxis, most of whom had "allergies" and 25% had asthma. Their categorization of "allergies" was unusual in that they included diseases such as urticaria and polyarthritis, thus calling into question the validity of this observation. Idsoe and colleagues[10] reported on a large series of 151 patients with fatal penicillin anaphylaxis "based on available medical literature." They characterized these patients according to the presence of "constitutional allergies" into bronchial asthma (14%), "others or unspecified types" (10%), and rhinitis in less than 1%; however, in greater than 50% of cases, data to determine allergies were not available. These authors actually recommended that, in patients with "constitutional allergies," penicillin treatment be used only in cases "not manageable by other antibiotics," a practice that has never been adopted. Thus, whether asthma or other atopic diseases are truly associated with penicillin anaphylaxis is not clear based on the literature.

In contrast with the association of mastocytosis and hymenoptera venom allergy in several studies, the role of drugs as triggers for anaphylaxis (IgE-mediated and non-IgE-mediated) in patients with mastocytosis is not as robust.[11] The most commonly implicated agents are opioids, NSAIDs, and muscle relaxants, and perioperative anaphylaxis can sometimes be the presenting manifestation. Conversely, in patients presenting with drug allergy, association with underlying mast cell disease has not been typically described.

Medications Exacerbating Anaphylaxis

Some anaphylactic reactions are contingent on the presence of obligate cofactors, which has led to the premise that some allergens elicit reactions only in the context of these amplifying factors and are otherwise tolerated without incident.[12] This finding is best described in exercise-induced anaphylaxis with foods as cofactors but also NSAIDs. With respect to drug-induced anaphylaxis, the best described of these augmentation factors are co-administered medications.

β-Blockade can augment mediator release in the setting of both IgE-mediated and non-IgE-mediated anaphylaxis. In addition, therapy may impede treatment effectiveness with epinephrine. In a case control study, the use of β-blockers significantly enhanced the risk for anaphylactic reactions to radiocontrast media (RCM), and these were more likely to be severe and treatment refractory.[13]

Angiotensin-converting enzyme inhibitors (ACE-Is) and angiotensin receptor blockers (ARBs) potentially increase severity of anaphylaxis by blocking the compensatory response to hypotension induced by angiotensin-2 activity. In addition, ACE-Is compromise the host ability to degrade bradykinin. In the cohort reported by Banerji and colleagues,[7] ACE-Is were among the most frequently prescribed medications at baseline.

A recent review of a German anaphylaxis database suggested that the combined use of β-blockers and ACE-Is modestly but significantly increases the risk for severe anaphylaxis.[14] In a murine model, the investigators showed the combination enhanced mast cell mediator release, especially in the setting of otherwise inadequate IgE receptor cross-linking. This phenomenon is clinically relevant because of frequent coprescription of these drug classes.

The role of ACE-Is in anaphylaxis has received a great deal of attention because it relates to immunotherapy, in particular, venom immunotherapy (VIT). Case reports have suggested an increased risk of anaphylaxis in patients taking ACE-Is who receive VIT. However, a recent report by Stoevesandt and colleagues[15] in a large group (n = 743) of patients treated with VIT did not show an increased risk of reactions in the 11.7% of patients who were maintained on an ACE-I during VIT. Thus, this area remains controversial.

Proton pump inhibitors (PPIs) have also been linked with drug-induced anaphylaxis in hospitalized patients, perhaps by interfering with the digestion, resulting in the persistence of allergenic proteins during gastric transit.[16]

PATHOGENESIS AND MECHANISMS

Drug-induced anaphylaxis can occur via both IgE-dependent and non-IgE-dependent pathways. Regarding IgE-dependent anaphylaxis, most drugs are too small to elicit an immune response and are thought to act as haptens or prohaptens in order to be immunogenic. Non-IgE-mediated anaphylaxis can be clinically indistinguishable from IgE-mediated anaphylaxis. Many mechanisms may result in non-IgE-mediated drug-induced anaphylaxis, including direct IgE-independent mast cell activation, complement activation, and kallikrein activation. Finally, drug-induced anaphylaxis can also occur because of contaminants. A range of catastrophic anaphylactic reactions to heparin contaminated with oversulfated chondroitin resulted in 80 deaths in the United States and Germany in 2007.[17]

CLINICAL FEATURES OF DRUG-INDUCED ANAPHYLAXIS

Drug-induced anaphylaxis has similar clinical manifestations as other forms of anaphylaxis. The most common manifestations of anaphylaxis are cutaneous with generalized urticaria and angioedema; however, respiratory, cardiovascular, gastrointestinal, and other symptoms may also occur. Biphasic and protracted cases of anaphylaxis also occur with drug-induced anaphylaxis with varying incidence rates due to drugs ranging from 0% to 10%.[18,19]

Vocal Cord Dysfunction Can Mimic Drug Anaphylaxis

Although some specialists are familiar with vocal cord dysfunction (VCD), most health care providers are unaware of this entity. Furthermore, the literature on VCD is primarily in relation to its presentation as "asthma"; however, many patients labeled with drug-induced "anaphylaxis" or "anaphylactic shock" actually have VCD. Patients with drug-associated VCD may have several symptoms, but the most severe symptoms relate to a sense of "throat swelling." This "swelling" occurs in the absence of objectively documented orofacial angioedema. In the authors' experience, many patients with drug-associated VCD will report subjective lip or tongue swelling, but this is not confirmed by health care providers despite that some family members may report seeing some "swelling." Many patients with drug-associated VCD report similar reactions to multiple different drugs. Challenge with the culprit drug followed by laryngoscopy is the best way to confirm a diagnosis.[20]

EVALUATION AND TREATMENT OF DRUG-INDUCED ANAPHYLAXIS

The management of drug-induced anaphylaxis is rife with unanswered questions. **Box 2** outlines unmet needs in diagnosis as well as treatment.

Initial Management of Anaphylaxis in the Acute Setting

Diagnosis and management

The diagnosis of drug-induced anaphylaxis remains a major problem in clinical practice. In most cases, a diagnosis can be made based on the clinical presentation. However, in cases where the diagnosis is less clear, confirmation of mediator release can be helpful (if positive). Total serum tryptase is the most widely used laboratory test to confirm anaphylaxis and is optimally obtained within 1 to 2 hours of onset of symptoms. Because some anaphylaxis patients may have normal values acutely,

---

Box 2
Unmet needs in drug-induced anaphylaxis

- Accurate epidemiologic data due to failure to differentiate between immunologic and nonimmunologic reactions, heterogeneity in study populations, and methodologies

- Identify host risk factors (genetic background, metabolism) and drug characteristics (metabolites and reactive groups) participating in hypersensitivity reactions

- Expanded standardized skin test reagents for medications other than penicillin

- Lack of an optimal, standardized laboratory test to confirm the diagnosis of an anaphylaxis episode

- Discrimination between allergen sensitization versus true risk for anaphylaxis

- Distinguishing subsets of patients at increased risk of fatal reactions

- Long-term reliability of negative skin tests and drug challenges

studies evaluating sting-induced anaphylaxis have suggested a relative increase greater than 135% of the baseline value to improve diagnosis.[21] Treatment of drug-induced anaphylaxis is similar to other forms of anaphylaxis.

Follow-Up Management After Resolution of the Acute Episode

A minority of patients with drug-induced anaphylaxis is discharged from the ED with epinephrine or undergo evaluation by an allergist in the subsequent year (8% referrals in the study by Banerji and colleagues[7]). Follow-up is crucial because, as indicated by epidemiologic studies, education regarding anaphylaxis is important in anticipation of potential future events.

In addition, there are relevant public health perspectives of interest. There is a clear need to increase drug allergy testing to reduce unnecessary avoidance of medications caused by presumed allergy. With regard to antibiotic allergy in particular, overdiagnosis is an issue for both adults and children and may contribute to the development of resistance by unnecessary use of broad-spectrum antibiotics. For instance, preoperative evaluation by an allergist with penicillin skin testing was demonstrated to be effective in decreasing the unnecessary perioperative administration of prophylactic vancomycin.[22] Patients with a label of penicillin "allergy" have recently been shown to have an increased risk of vancomycin-resistant *Enterococcus*, *Clostridium difficile*, and methicillin-resistant *Staphylococcus aureus* infections.[23] However, tests with improved diagnostic accuracy for drugs other than penicillin remain an unmet need.

The clinical management relies heavily on clinical history, with correlations to timing of medication exposure and associated symptoms. Diagnostic tools have primarily focused on IgE-mediated anaphylaxis with implementation of skin prick test (SPT) and intradermal drug tests (IDT) and, rarely, drug-specific IgE testing when available.

In vivo testing (skin tests)

The technique for performing skin testing to drugs is extensively discussed in the Drug Allergy Practice Parameter.[24] It is critical to understand that with the exception of a few medications (eg, penicillin) a negative skin test to most drugs does not equate with the absence of allergy. For patients with histories of drug-induced anaphylaxis, SPT are typically performed with the undiluted drug. If SPT is negative, IDT are performed with sequential dilutions starting as low as 1/10,000 up to 1/10 (or a nonirritating concentration) on the volar aspect of the forearm. The authors typically recommend aiming for a 5 × 5-mm wheal with IDT. There is no uniform agreement on what constitutes a positive skin test response, but most experts agree that it is defined by the size of the wheal, which should be 3 mm or greater than that of the negative control for either prick/puncture or intradermal tests.[24] It is generally advised to perform testing at least 6 weeks after the episode to avoid any possible refractory period in which testing may be negative. When testing is indeterminate, replicate testing should be performed.

In vitro testing

Serum-specific Immunoglobulin E assays Allergen-specific IgE testing is available for numerous drugs, including β-lactams, cefaclor, bovine gelatin, and insulin, and in general has lower specificity and sensitivity than skin testing. The diagnostic accuracy for nearly all commercially available drug-specific IgE tests has not been established.

Basophil activation testing The diagnostic role of the basophil activation testing (BAT) has been gaining attention recently. This flow cytometry–based cellular assay measures the activation of basophils on allergen stimulation using CD63 and

CD203c (markers of degranulation); these may detect IgE-mediated or non-IgE-mediated hypersensitivity. Commercially available BATs do not have established diagnostic accuracy.

Drug Challenges

Drug challenges are primarily indicated in patients wherein the clinical suspicion is low for true drug allergy. In a patient with a likely diagnosis of drug-induced anaphylaxis, drug challenges should not be performed to the culprit drug. Negative skin tests to most implicated drugs lack the negative predictive value to recommend drug challenges in the setting of a reliable history.

However, drug challenges may be helpful to find alternatives to an implicated drug. In addition, in a patient labeled with drug "anaphylaxis," in which the clinical reaction is not really anaphylaxis, a drug challenge can be considered, if the likelihood of true drug allergy is low. Patients with drug-associated VCD benefit from drug challenge in conjunction with laryngoscopy. In patients who are deemed appropriate to undergo drug challenges, reactions occur in less than 15%. In a retrospective review of drug challenges at the authors' institution, some of whom were labeled with "anaphylaxis," only 1 of 114 patients developed a mild, delayed skin reaction in a series of 123 total challenges.[25] Although the traditional drug challenge consists of stepwise graduations starting at 1/100 to 1/1000 of the final dose, a recent review suggests that a one-step or two-step test dose strategy (as opposed to a multistep challenge) might be appropriate and safe.[26] **Box 3** provides clinical scenarios wherein drug challenges may be indicated.

If a patient with reported medication hypersensitivity is found to be nonallergic following evaluation, the medical record should be accordingly amended to reflect this status change. Documentation of tolerance to a related medication class in a drug-allergic patient is similarly important (for example, tolerance of cephalosporins in a penicillin-allergic patient).

Desensitization Protocols

Rapid desensitization is used clinically to prevent the occurrence of anaphylaxis (and other severe, mostly IgE-mediated) allergic reactions in patients who are sensitized to the particular medication, when substitutions with an alternative are not possible. It implies a temporary induction of tolerance that is maintained for the duration of exposure to the drug. Beginning with a low dose (~10,000-fold less than therapeutic), increasing amounts are administered every 15 to 20 minutes over a period of several

---

Box 3
Indications for drug challenges in drug-induced anaphylaxis

- Challenge with culprit drug
  - To exclude drug allergy in patients whose history is not suggestive of drug allergy or anaphylaxis
  - To exclude drug allergy in patients with negative penicillin skin tests
  - To confirm VCD in a suspect patient
- Challenge with alternative drug
  - To provide evidence of tolerance to potentially cross-reacting drugs
  - To distinguish selective responders from cross-reactors, for instance, in cases of β-lactam or NSAID anaphylaxis

hours until a therapeutic dose is achieved. Liu and colleagues[27] and Sancho-Serra and colleagues[28] have reported on drug desensitization outcomes using a 3-bag, 12-step desensitization protocol that was developed, partly based on an in vitro model of mast cell desensitization. The anergy thus effected in mast cells and basophils is transient, and the protocol must be repeated each time treatment is interrupted. The principles of these rapid desensitization protocols can be applied to numerous medications, including antibiotics, chemotherapeutics, and monoclonal antibodies.

Medication-specific desensitization protocols are available for several drug classes and follow a general theme of doubling doses at short intervals. The aforementioned Drug Allergy Practice Parameter has several desensitization protocols.[24]

Specific Drugs Causing Anaphylaxis

Nonsteroidal anti-inflammatory drugs

NSAIDs are among the most common class of medications implicated in adult hypersensitivity drug reactions (responsible for 21% to 25% of reported adverse drug events), and ibuprofen accounts for up to 30% of documented episodes. Numerous hypersensitivity reactions exist with NSAIDs. Some of these reactions occur with the entire class (eg, aspirin exacerbated respiratory disease) and others are drug-specific.

NSAID-induced anaphylaxis is typically a drug-specific reaction.[29,30] The most frequently responsible NSAIDs are pyrazolones, diclofenac, and propionic acid derivatives. Although aspirin has often been reported to cause anaphylaxis, there are no convincing cases reported in the literature of true anaphylaxis from aspirin.[31]

An IgE-mediated mechanism has been suggested based on tolerance to other strong COX-1 inhibitors. Although risk factors have not been delineated, gastric acid suppression may be a factor in the induction of IgE-mediated diclofenac allergy based on a murine model, wherein only mice receiving diclofenac under gastric acid suppression developed IgE in a dose-dependent fashion.[32]

Other than pyrazolones,[33] skin tests in IgE-sensitized patients have typically given negative results, implicating various activation and haptenation processes in the genesis of IgE hypersensitivity to NSAIDs. Similarly, specific IgE has not been consistently detected in presumed type 1 reactions. Diagnostic accuracy of commercially available BAT tests for NSAID-anaphylaxis has not been established.

Drug challenge to a nonstructurally related NSAID has been shown to be a safe and effective method to show tolerance to other NSAIDs in patients with NSAID anaphylaxis. Initial doses varied considerably by drug, ranging from 10% to 50% of the drug with subsequent doses being administered every 1 to 2 hours for 2 to 4 doses (**Table 1**).

After tolerance to another NSAID or acetaminophen is determined, the culprit NSAID and structurally related NSAIDs should be strictly avoided. Although an IgE-mediated mechanism is suspected, validated protocols for NSAID desensitization in patients with anaphylaxis are lacking.

Antibiotics

Penicillins Among all causes of drug-induced anaphylaxis, penicillin in the 1960s and 1970s was purported to be the most common cause in the United States, with β-lactam antibiotics allegedly responsible for 400 to 800 fatal anaphylactic episodes per year. More recently, in a UK database of anaphylaxis, amoxicillin was the single most common cause of antibiotic-induced reactions (13 of 102 total cases).[34]

The β-lactam ring of penicillin is unstable and opens to conjugate with carrier proteins to form the major allergenic determinant (penicilloyl polylysine). However,

Table 1
Alternative nonsteroidal anti-inflammatory drug challenge protocol for nonsteroidal anti-inflammatory drug anaphylaxis

Drug	Doses (mg)	Challenge Interval (min)
Celecoxib	50, 100, 200	60
Diclofenac	25, 50	120
Ibuprofen	50, 150, 250, 600	60
Meloxicam	7.5, 15	60

Data from Quiralte J, Blanco C, Delgado J, et al. Challenge-based clinical patterns of 223 Spanish patients with nonsteroidal anti-inflammatory-drug-induced-reactions. J Investig Allergol Clin Immunol 2007;17(3):182–8.

IgE antibodies to β-lactam drugs are heterogeneous, and IgE binding sites of semisynthetic penicillins may target the R-side chain. Most of this data originated from Spain and involves the aminopenicillins.[35]

Clinical history alone is a poor predictor of reactivity to penicillin. Several studies, although not perfectly comparable, have demonstrated that the IgE response to penicillin decreases with time, with approximately 10% of patients per year losing skin test sensitivity.[36,37] Penicillin skin testing is an excellent diagnostic tool with the greatest experience of any drug tested. The major determinant of penicillin (benzylpenicilloyl polylysine [PRE-PEN]) is commercially available, without need for dilution for skin testing. Both American and European guidelines recommend the use of major and a minor determinant mixture (MDM), which contains penicillin G, penicilloate, penilloate, and/or penicilloylamine. Only penicillin G is commercially available in the United States but requires dilution for skin testing. Penicillin skin testing using both major and MDM has excellent negative predictive value, even in cases of anaphylaxis. Although it has been reported that MDM positivity is associated with anaphylaxis,[38] this has not been well documented. Levine and Zolov[39] stated that MDM-positive patients seem to be at "the highest risk of immediate (including anaphylactic) allergic reaction." This conclusion was based on prior studies in which anaphylactic reactions were associated with penicillin G reactivity,[40] and their own observations that 2 MDM-positive patients reacted during an attempted (and undefined) desensitization procedure. Because MDM contains penicillin G among others, it is not known which of these reagins (if any) has a higher predictive value for anaphylaxis.

A recent study by Macy and Ngor[41] showed a negative predictive value of 96% to 99% using PRE-PEN and penicillin G (without MDM) followed by amoxicillin challenge in 500 consecutive patients with penicillin allergy. The caveat of this study is that these patients had remote reactions and less than 3% had histories of anaphylaxis. Therefore, caution should be exercised in challenging patients with histories of true penicillin anaphylaxis after negative skin tests without MDM. If the history was recent, one may still wish to avoid penicillin or perform a desensitization if testing cannot be performed with MDM. In vitro testing for specific IgE has no significant role in the evaluation of penicillin anaphylaxis.

Clavulanic acid has also been implicated in immediate reactions to formulations in which it is combined with amoxicillin, and, in the setting of a consistent clinical history, should also be tested when penicillin allergy evaluation is negative. One small study recommended IDT with amoxicillin-clavulanic acid at 20 mg/mL (from the intravenous preparation, not available in the United States) or clavulanic acid itself at 1 mg/mL.[42]

Positive skin testing to penicillin generally mandates alternative antibiotic use; however, if there are no other agents indicated, desensitization procedures may be used and are well-established for penicillin.[43] The procedure is typically successful, although 30% of patients tend to develop minor cutaneous reactions.

Other β-Lactams

Cephalosporins

Anaphylactic reactions to cephalosporins are rare. Macy and Contreras[44] recently reported only 5 of 901,908 oral courses or 8 of 487,630 courses. The incidence of severe anaphylactic reactions to cephalosporins was more than half the rate to penicillins but accounted for 12.3% of all cases from the French Allergy Vigilance Network.[45]

Reactions to cephalosporins are most often side chain specific as opposed to being directed at the β-lactam ring. Skin testing to cephalosporins using concentrations of 2 mg/mL has been used in patients with immediate reactions to cephalosporins and was positive in 72% of patients; however, its accuracy in patients with cephalosporin anaphylaxis is unclear.[46] In the aforementioned severe anaphylaxis study, ~83% with cephalosporin anaphylaxis had positive skin tests, with 58.5% positive with SPT.

Most patients with a history of cephalosporin allergy seem to tolerate other structurally unrelated cephalosporins. If necessary, challenges to alternative medications may be appropriate using cephalosporins with different R1 or R2 side chains than the original culprit drug. **Table 2** categorizes β-lactams based on identical R1 and R2 side chains.

Table 2
β-Lactams with identical R1 side chains

First-Generation and Second-Generation Cephalosporins and Penicillins[a]		
Identical Aminobenzyl Group	Identical Aminobenzyl Group	Common Methylene Group in R1 Side Chain
Amoxicillin	Ampicillin	Benzyl penicillin
Cefadroxil	Cephalexin	Cephalothin
Cefatrizine	Cefaclor	
Cefprozil	Cephradine	
	Cephaloglycin	
	Loracarbef	

Third-Generation and Fourth-Generation Cephalosporins and Aztreonam[b]	
Common Methoxymino Group	Identical R1 Side Chain
Ceftriaxone	Ceftazidime
Cefuroxime	Aztreonam
Cefotaxime	
Cefepime	

Cephalosporins with Identical R2 Side Chains[c]					
Cephalexin	Cefotaxime	Cefuroxime	Cefotetan	Cefaclor	Ceftibutin
Cefadroxil	Cephalothin	Cefoxitin	Cefamandole	Loracarbef	Ceftizoxime
Cephradine	Cephaloglycin		Cefmetazole		
			Cefpiramide		

Clinically significant with respect to generation of allergenic epitopes.
 [a] Includes thiazolyl and phenylglycyl side chains similar to penicillins.
 [b] Based on an aminothiazole-oxime moiety; do not cross-react with penicillins.
 [c] Limited and vague associations with allergenicity and cross-reactive responses.

Carbapenems

The frequency of reported HSR to carbapenems is estimated to be approximately 2% to 3%, and anaphylactic reactions are rare. Skin testing has not been well studied in this class of antibiotic and the negative predictive value is largely unknown. Chen and colleagues[47] diagnosed a case of IgE-mediated anaphylaxis to imipenem-cilastatin based on positive SPT at a concentration of 1 mg/mL to each component, and positive serum-specific IgE. Successful desensitization regimens to both imipenem and meropenem have been described in isolated case reports.[48,49]

Monobactams

Aztreonam is generally less immunogenic than other β-lactams because haptens are less likely to be formed. In single cases, skin testing with native aztreonam (2 mg/mL) was nonirritating and established a diagnosis of immediate hypersensitivity.[50,51] Anaphylaxis to aztreonam has rarely been reported.[52]

Cross-reactivity among β-lactams

Another common clinical conundrum is the administration of potentially cross-reactive medications in patients labeled with allergy to β-lactam antibiotics. Cross-reactivity is frequent among penicillins as well as among cephalosporins. Overall, most recent studies describe much lower rates of potential cross-reactivity between different classes of β-lactams. Romano and colleagues[53–55] have evaluated patients with penicillin anaphylaxis and found that negative skin testing to cephalosporins or carbapenems, followed by graded challenge, is well tolerated. This group has also evaluated cephalosporin anaphylactic patients and found that after negative skin tests and challenge, 75% will tolerate penicillins and greater than 95% can tolerate aztreonam, imipenem/cilastin, and meropenem.[56] There are no comparable data for patients with anaphylaxis to carbapenems or aztreonam (given their rarity), but a similar approach of skin testing and challenge to other β-lactams seems reasonable.

Non-β-lactam antibiotics

Anaphylaxis to sulfonamides or trimethoprim is rare with case reports showing positive skin tests at nonirritating concentrations.[57] Anaphylaxis to macrolides is also rare but case reports exist showing positive skin tests and successful desensitization.[58]

Allergic reactions to quinolones are increasing, including anaphylaxis. In the aforementioned French severe anaphylaxis study, quinolones were responsible for 9% of severe antibiotic anaphylaxis.[45] A recent study of 66 patients confirmed with immediate hypersensitivity to fluoroquinolones showed that ~75% had anaphylaxis, with moxifloxacin being the most common culprit, followed by ciprofloxacin.[59] Most authors have found skin testing to quinolones to cause false positives, and therefore, it is not recommended in the evaluation of patients with suspected quinolone allergy. Patients with anaphylaxis to one quinolone may tolerate others via graded challenge but there are no general rules to predict cross-reactivity among different quinolones.[60] Another unresolved issue is that quinolones can cause generalized pruritus, flushing, and even anaphylaxis after the first dose, likely because of high intracellular penetration and nonspecific histamine release.[61]

Vancomycin is a glycopeptide best known for causing the "red man syndrome": a pseudoallergic reaction resulting from direct mast cell stimulation, associated with rapid intravenous administration and characterized by flushing and pruritus, although more severe reactions including hypotension and muscle spasms may develop. Prolonging the infusion time more than 60 minutes, pretreatment with antihistamines, and avoidance of concomitant narcotics are typically helpful; however, rapid induction of drug tolerance protocols have been used successfully in patients who are refractory to these measures.[62] IgE-mediated reactions are rarely reported,[63] and skin testing using vancomycin at 0.05 mg/mL is nonirritating.[64] Teicoplanin is another glycopeptide that does not cause histamine release even at rapid infusion rates; anaphylaxis has rarely been reported with this medication.[65]

Radiocontrast media

Reactions to intravenous contrast were previously deemed non-IgE-mediated (through activation of complement) with systemic reactions reported in 3.8% to 12.1% of patients receiving ionic RCM. These events remain a significant threat despite the advent of nonionic, low osmolar contrast media, albeit at a lower rate of 0.7% to 3.1%.[66] However, both ionic and nonionic RCM may trigger anaphylaxis that has been postulated to be IgE-mediated.

Anaphylaxis to gadolinium agents used in MRI may also occur, although much less frequently than reactions to aforementioned RCM. Undiluted SPT and IDT of gadolinium at 1:10 dilution has been shown to be helpful in 2 patients (nonirritating in 10 controls); however, more data are needed.[67]

A recent study from Korea analyzed 104 cases of RCM-induced anaphylaxis: 85% had cardiovascular symptoms, 66% had cutaneous manifestations, and 48% had respiratory symptoms.[66] Most symptoms occurred within minutes of exposure. Older age and multiple previous exposures to RCM were more likely to have anaphylaxis associated with hypotension. Fatalities have been reported even after the introduction of nonionic media, with most cases lacking predictable risk factors.[68] Despite common misperceptions, RCM reactions are not due to iodine nor are they related to shellfish allergy; thus, fish or shellfish allergy does not confer higher risk to RCM reactions of any severity nor is the inverse true.[69]

Recognition of the potential for IgE-mediated RCM reactions has resulted in revisiting the role of skin testing in evaluation, with undiluted SPT followed by IDT at a dilution of 1:10.[70] A large prospective study of 1048 patients who underwent IDT at 1:10 concentration found only one patient with a positive reaction, indicating this concentration is nonirritating.[71] The rate of positive skin tests in patients with immediate RCM reactions varies by study, but does seem to be higher in those with more severe reactions. In the Korean study of RCM anaphylaxis, 65% of 51 patients who underwent skin tests had positive results.[66] Skin test positivity was even higher in those with anaphylactic shock (82%). Positive skin tests may also vary with time with less than 25% positive more than 6 months after the reaction.[70] The negative predictive value of these tests is still not entirely clear. A small study from Spain showed that 2 patients with RCM anaphylaxis who were skin test negative had positive challenges to that agent.[72] Thus, the precise role of skin testing in the evaluation of RCM anaphylaxis is still evolving, but it certainly could be considered in the evaluation of these patients.

Premedication in patients at high risk for an RCM reaction using corticosteroids and antihistamines was a well-established management plan for reactions to ionic RCM agents, as shown by Greenberger and colleagues.[73] Since then, different studies have shown mixed results with varying rates of breakthrough reactions using heterogeneous premedication protocols.[74,75] A systematic review concluded that randomized controlled trials are lacking to support the efficacy of premedication in subjects with allergic reactions to RCM.[76] Doubling the premedication period (ie, starting up to 31 hours before with every 6-hour dosing of prednisone) may lessen the severity of breakthrough reactions (A. Ditto, personal communication, 2015).

Changing the type of contrast agent has been recommended and seems reasonable, especially if there is a potential for an IgE-mediated reaction. A recent case report described successful desensitization to the nonionic RCM iodixanol, with the background of recurrent reactions despite premedication.[77]

Opioids

Most reactions to opioids are secondary to nonimmunologic induction of histamine release (pseudoallergic). Pruritus is a frequent symptom; flushing, urticaria, and mild hypotension may also occur. The most common offenders are the low-potency opiates (meperidine, codeine, and morphine). High-potency opioids such as fentanyl and hydromorphone are less likely to cause histamine release. IgE-mediated anaphylaxis to opioids has rarely been reported.[78] SPTs to opiates cannot differentiate opiate allergic patients from controls, likely because of nonspecific mast cell release, suggesting drug challenge is necessary.

Heparin

Delayed reactions to subcutaneously administered heparins are more commonly seen than immediate hypersensitivity reactions. Anaphylactic reactions to heparin (including low-molecular-weight heparins) are extremely rare and knowledge is mostly confined to case reports. Cross-reactivity among heparins in cases of anaphylaxis has been reported but data are sparse.[79] Immediate skin tests, together with drug challenges, are indicated as reliable diagnostic tools in evaluation of immediate heparin allergy to find alternative agents. It has been recommended to use undiluted heparin solutions for SPT and 1:10 dilution for IDT.[80]

Proton pump inhibitors

PPIs are increasingly being reported as causing severe drug reactions, including anaphylaxis; however, given their frequent usage, anaphylactic reactions are still rare. Data on skin testing to PPIs have recently been reviewed and nonirritating doses for SPT concentrations are as follows: 40 mg/mL for omeprazole, esomeprazole, and pantoprazole; 30 mg/mL for lansoprazole; and 20 mg/mL for rabeprazole.[81] IDT can be performed at a 1:10 dilution. A recent study reported the accuracy of SPT and IDT for the diagnosis of immediate hypersensitivity to PPIs, with positive skin tests (in 12 of 53 patients) appearing to correlate with severity of the reaction.[82] Oral drug challenges were performed in this study and suggested good negative predictive value (92%); however, only 1 of 9 severe reactors underwent challenge and thus severe reactors were excluded from this accuracy analysis. Cross-reactivity among PPIs is quite variable and not consistent across studies.

REFERENCES

1. Wood RA, Camargo CA Jr, Lieberman P, et al. Anaphylaxis in America: the prevalence and characteristics of anaphylaxis in the United States. J Allergy Clin Immunol 2014;133(2):461–7.
2. Huang F, Chawla K, Jarvinen KM, et al. Anaphylaxis in a New York City pediatric emergency department: triggers, treatments, and outcomes. J Allergy Clin Immunol 2012;129(1):162–8.e1–3.
3. Jerschow E, Lin RY, Scaperotti MM, et al. Fatal anaphylaxis in the United States, 1999–2010: temporal patterns and demographic associations. J Allergy Clin Immunol 2014;134(6):1318–28.e7.
4. Liew WK, Williamson E, Tang ML. Anaphylaxis fatalities and admissions in Australia. J Allergy Clin Immunol 2009;123(2):434–42.

5. Clark S, Wei W, Rudders SA, et al. Risk factors for severe anaphylaxis in patients receiving anaphylaxis treatment in US emergency departments and hospitals. J Allergy Clin Immunol 2014;134(5):1125–30.
6. Brown SG, Stone SF, Fatovich DM, et al. Anaphylaxis: clinical patterns, mediator release, and severity. J Allergy Clin Immunol 2013;132(5):1141–9.e5.
7. Banerji A, Rudders S, Clark S, et al. Retrospective study of drug-induced anaphylaxis treated in the emergency department or hospital: patient characteristics, management, and 1-year follow-up. J Allergy Clin Immunol Pract 2014;2(1):46–51.
8. Vadas P, Perelman B, Liss G. Platelet-activating factor, histamine, and tryptase levels in human anaphylaxis. J Allergy Clin Immunol 2013;131(1):144–9.
9. Bertelsen K, Dalgaard JB. Death due to penicillin. 16 Danish cases with autopsies. Nord Med 1965;73:173–7 [in Swedish].
10. Idsoe O, Guthe T, Willcox RR, et al. Nature and extent of penicillin side-reactions, with particular reference to fatalities from anaphylactic shock. Bull World Health Organ 1968;38(2):159–88.
11. Brockow K, Bonadonna P. Drug allergy in mast cell disease. Curr Opin Allergy Clin Immunol 2012;12(4):354–60.
12. Wolbing F, Fischer J, Koberle M, et al. About the role and underlying mechanisms of cofactors in anaphylaxis. Allergy 2013;68(9):1085–92.
13. Lang DM, Alpern MB, Visintainer PF, et al. Elevated risk of anaphylactoid reaction from radiographic contrast media is associated with both beta-blocker exposure and cardiovascular disorders. Arch Intern Med 1993;153(17):2033–40.
14. Nassiri M, Babina M, Dolle S, et al. Ramipril and metoprolol intake aggravate human and murine anaphylaxis: evidence for direct mast cell priming. J Allergy Clin Immunol 2015;135(2):491–9.
15. Stoevesandt J, Hain J, Stolze I, et al. Angiotensin-converting enzyme inhibitors do not impair the safety of Hymenoptera venom immunotherapy build-up phase. Clin Exp Allergy 2014;44(5):747–55.
16. Ramirez E, Cabanas R, Laserna LS, et al. Proton pump inhibitors are associated with hypersensitivity reactions to drugs in hospitalized patients: a nested case-control in a retrospective cohort study. Clin Exp Allergy 2013;43(3):344–52.
17. Kishimoto TK, Viswanathan K, Ganguly T, et al. Contaminated heparin associated with adverse clinical events and activation of the contact system. N Engl J Med 2008;358(23):2457–67.
18. Lee S, Bellolio MF, Hess EP, et al. Predictors of biphasic reactions in the emergency department for patients with anaphylaxis. J Allergy Clin Immunol Pract 2014;2(3):281–7.
19. Ellis AK, Day JH. Incidence and characteristics of biphasic anaphylaxis: a prospective evaluation of 103 patients. Ann Allergy Asthma Immunol 2007;98(1):64–9.
20. Khan DA. Treating patients with multiple drug allergies. Ann Allergy Asthma Immunol 2013;110(1):2–6.
21. Borer-Reinhold M, Haeberli G, Bitzenhofer M, et al. An increase in serum tryptase even below 11.4 ng/mL may indicate a mast cell-mediated hypersensitivity reaction: a prospective study in Hymenoptera venom allergic patients. Clin Exp Allergy 2011;41(12):1777–83.
22. Park M, Markus P, Matesic D, et al. Safety and effectiveness of a preoperative allergy clinic in decreasing vancomycin use in patients with a history of penicillin allergy. Ann Allergy Asthma Immunol 2006;97(5):681–7.
23. Macy E, Contreras R. Health care use and serious infection prevalence associated with penicillin "allergy" in hospitalized patients: a cohort study. J Allergy Clin Immunol 2014;133(3):790–6.

24. Joint Task Force on Practice Parameters, American Academy of Allergy, Asthma and Immunology, American College of Allergy, Asthma and Immunology, et al. Drug allergy: an updated practice parameter. Ann Allergy Asthma Immunol 2010;105(4):259–73.
25. Kao L, Rajan J, Roy L, et al. Adverse reactions during drug challenges: a single US institution's experience. Ann Allergy Asthma Immunol 2013;110(2):86–91.e1.
26. Iammatteo M, Blumenthal KG, Saff R, et al. Safety and outcomes of test doses for the evaluation of adverse drug reactions: a 5-year retrospective review. J Allergy Clin Immunol Pract 2014;2:768–74.
27. Liu A, Fanning L, Chong H, et al. Desensitization regimens for drug allergy: state of the art in the 21st century. Clin Exp Allergy 2011;41(12):1679–89.
28. Sancho-Serra MC, Simarro M, Castells M. Rapid IgE desensitization is antigen specific and impairs early and late mast cell responses targeting FcεRI internalization. Eur J Immunol 2011;41(4):1004–13.
29. Quiralte J, Blanco C, Castillo R, et al. Intolerance to nonsteroidal antiinflammatory drugs: results of controlled drug challenges in 98 patients. J Allergy Clin Immunol 1996;98(3):678–85.
30. Quiralte J, Blanco C, Delgado J, et al. Challenge-based clinical patterns of 223 Spanish patients with nonsteroidal anti-inflammatory-drug-induced-reactions. J Investig Allergol Clin Immunol 2007;17(3):182–8.
31. White AA, Stevenson DD, Woessner KM, et al. Approach to patients with aspirin hypersensitivity and acute cardiovascular emergencies. Allergy Asthma Proc 2013;34(2):138–42.
32. Riemer AB, Gruber S, Pali-Scholl I, et al. Suppression of gastric acid increases the risk of developing immunoglobulin E-mediated drug hypersensitivity: human diclofenac sensitization and a murine sensitization model. Clin Exp Allergy 2010;40(3):486–93.
33. Himly M, Jahn-Schmid B, Pittertschatscher K, et al. IgE-mediated immediate-type hypersensitivity to the pyrazolone drug propyphenazone. J Allergy Clin Immunol 2003;111(4):882–8.
34. Gonzalez-Perez A, Aponte Z, Vidaurre CF, et al. Anaphylaxis epidemiology in patients with and patients without asthma: a United Kingdom database review. J Allergy Clin Immunol 2010;125(5):1098–104.e1.
35. Blanca M, Vega JM, Garcia J, et al. Allergy to penicillin with good tolerance to other penicillins; study of the incidence in subjects allergic to beta-lactams. Clin Exp Allergy 1990;20(5):475–81.
36. Sullivan TJ, Wedner HJ, Shatz GS, et al. Skin testing to detect penicillin allergy. J Allergy Clin Immunol 1981;68(3):171–80.
37. Blanca M, Torres MJ, Garcia JJ, et al. Natural evolution of skin test sensitivity in patients allergic to beta-lactam antibiotics. J Allergy Clin Immunol 1999;103(5 Pt 1):918–24.
38. Gadde J, Spence M, Wheeler B, et al. Clinical experience with penicillin skin testing in a large inner-city STD clinic. JAMA 1993;270(20):2456–63.
39. Levine BB, Zolov DM. Prediction of penicillin allergy by immunological tests. J Allergy 1969;43(4):231–44.
40. Siegel BB, Levine BB. Antigenic specificities of skin-sensitizing antibodies in sera from patients with immediate systemic allergic reactions to penicillin. J Allergy 1964;35:488–98.
41. Macy E, Ngor EW. Safely diagnosing clinically significant penicillin allergy using only penicilloyl-poly-lysine, penicillin, and oral amoxicillin. J Allergy Clin Immunol Pract 2013;1:258–63.

42. Sanchez-Morillas L, Perez-Ezquerra PR, Reano-Martos M, et al. Selective allergic reactions to clavulanic acid: a report of 9 cases. J Allergy Clin Immunol 2010; 126(1):177–9.
43. Wendel GD Jr, Stark BJ, Jamison RB, et al. Penicillin allergy and desensitization in serious infections during pregnancy. N Engl J Med 1985;312(19):1229–32.
44. Macy E, Contreras R. Adverse reactions associated with oral and parenteral use of cephalosporins: a retrospective population-based analysis. J Allergy Clin Immunol 2014.
45. Renaudin JM, Beaudouin E, Ponvert C, et al. Severe drug-induced anaphylaxis: analysis of 333 cases recorded by the Allergy Vigilance Network from 2002 to 2010. Allergy 2013;68(7):929–37.
46. Romano A, Gueant-Rodriguez RM, Viola M, et al. Diagnosing immediate reactions to cephalosporins. Clin Exp Allergy 2005;35(9):1234–42.
47. Chen Z, Baur X, Kutscha-Lissberg F, et al. IgE-mediated anaphylactic reaction to imipenem. Allergy 2000;55(1):92–3.
48. Wilson DL, Owens RC Jr, Zuckerman JB. Successful meropenem desensitization in a patient with cystic fibrosis. Ann Pharmacother 2003;37(10):1424–8.
49. Gorman SK, Zed PJ, Dhingra VK, et al. Rapid imipenem/cilastatin desensitization for multidrug-resistant acinetobacter pneumonia. Ann Pharmacother 2003;37(4): 513–6.
50. Perez Pimiento A, Gomez Martinez M, Minguez Mena A, et al. Aztreonam and ceftazidime: evidence of in vivo cross allergenicity. Allergy 1998;53(6):624–5.
51. de la Fuente Prieto R, Armentia Medina A, Sanchez Palla P, et al. Urticaria caused by sensitization to aztreonam. Allergy 1993;48(8):634–6.
52. Iglesias Cadarso A, Saez Jimenez SA, Vidal Pan C, et al. Aztreonam-induced anaphylaxis. Lancet 1990;336(8717):746–7.
53. Romano A, Gueant-Rodriguez RM, Viola M, et al. Cross-reactivity and tolerability of cephalosporins in patients with immediate hypersensitivity to penicillins. Ann Intern Med 2004;141(1):16–22.
54. Romano A, Viola M, Gueant-Rodriguez RM, et al. Imipenem in patients with immediate hypersensitivity to penicillins. N Engl J Med 2006;354(26):2835–7.
55. Romano A, Viola M, Gueant-Rodriguez RM, et al. Brief communication: tolerability of meropenem in patients with IgE-mediated hypersensitivity to penicillins. Ann Intern Med 2007;146(4):266–9.
56. Romano A, Gaeta F, Valluzzi RL, et al. IgE-mediated hypersensitivity to cephalosporins: cross-reactivity and tolerability of penicillins, monobactams, and carbapenems. J Allergy Clin Immunol 2010;126(5):994–9.
57. Bijl AM, Van der Klauw MM, Van Vliet AC, et al. Anaphylactic reactions associated with trimethoprim. Clin Exp Allergy 1998;28(4):510–2.
58. Swamy N, Laurie SA, Ruiz-Huidobro E, et al. Successful clarithromycin desensitization in a multiple macrolide-allergic patient. Ann Allergy Asthma Immunol 2010;105(6):489–90.
59. Blanca-Lopez N, Ariza A, Dona I, et al. Hypersensitivity reactions to fluoroquinolones: analysis of the factors involved. Clin Exp Allergy 2013;43(5):560–7.
60. Blanca-Lopez N, Andreu I, Torres Jaen MJ. Hypersensitivity reactions to quinolones. Curr Opin Allergy Clin Immunol 2011;11(4):285–91.
61. Kelesidis T, Fleisher J, Tsiodras S. Anaphylactoid reaction considered ciprofloxacin related: a case report and literature review. Clin Ther 2010;32(3):515–26.
62. Wong JT, Ripple RE, MacLean JA, et al. Vancomycin hypersensitivity: synergism with narcotics and "desensitization" by a rapid continuous intravenous protocol. J Allergy Clin Immunol 1994;94(2 Pt 1):189–94.

63. Knudsen JD, Pedersen M. IgE-mediated reaction to vancomycin and teicoplanin after treatment with vancomycin. Scand J Infect Dis 1992;24(3):395–6.
64. Empedrad R, Darter AL, Earl HS, et al. Nonirritating intradermal skin test concentrations for commonly prescribed antibiotics. J Allergy Clin Immunol 2003;112(3): 629–30.
65. Asero R. Teicoplanin-induced anaphylaxis. Allergy 2006;61(11):1370.
66. Kim MH, Lee SY, Lee SE, et al. Anaphylaxis to iodinated contrast media: clinical characteristics related with development of anaphylactic shock. PLoS One 2014; 9(6):e100154.
67. Galera C, Pur Ozygit L, Cavigioli S, et al. Gadoteridol-induced anaphylaxis—not a class allergy. Allergy 2010;65(1):132–4.
68. Palmiere C, Reggiani Bonetti L. Risk factors in fatal cases of anaphylaxis due to contrast media: a forensic evaluation. Int Arch Allergy Immunol 2014;164(4): 280–8.
69. Beaty AD, Lieberman PL, Slavin RG. Seafood allergy and radiocontrast media: are physicians propagating a myth? Am J Med 2008;121(2):158.e1–4.
70. Brockow K, Romano A, Aberer W, et al. Skin testing in patients with hypersensitivity reactions to iodinated contrast media—a European multicenter study. Allergy 2009;64(2):234–41.
71. Kim SH, Jo EJ, Kim MY, et al. Clinical value of radiocontrast media skin tests as a prescreening and diagnostic tool in hypersensitivity reactions. Ann Allergy Asthma Immunol 2013;110(4):258–62.
72. Salas M, Gomez F, Fernandez TD, et al. Diagnosis of immediate hypersensitivity reactions to radiocontrast media. Allergy 2013;68(9):1203–6.
73. Greenberger PA, Patterson R, Radin RC. Two pretreatment regimens for high-risk patients receiving radiographic contrast media. J Allergy Clin Immunol 1984; 74(4 Pt 1):540–3.
74. Freed KS, Leder RA, Alexander C, et al. Breakthrough adverse reactions to low-osmolar contrast media after steroid premedication. AJR Am J Roentgenol 2001;176(6):1389–92.
75. Davenport MS, Cohan RH, Caoili EM, et al. Repeat contrast medium reactions in premedicated patients: frequency and severity. Radiology 2009;253(2):372–9.
76. Tramer MR, von Elm E, Loubeyre P, et al. Pharmacological prevention of serious anaphylactic reactions due to iodinated contrast media: systematic review. BMJ 2006;333(7570):675.
77. Gandhi S, Litt D, Chandy M, et al. Successful rapid intravenous desensitization for radioiodine contrast allergy in a patient requiring urgent coronary angiography. J Allergy Clin Immunol Pract 2014;2(1):101–2.
78. Harle DG, Baldo BA, Coroneos NJ, et al. Anaphylaxis following administration of papaveretum. Case report: implication of IgE antibodies that react with morphine and codeine, and identification of an allergenic determinant. Anesthesiology 1989;71(4):489–94.
79. Gonzalez P, de la Sen ML, Venegas I, et al. Immediate hypersensitivity to heparins: a cross-reactivity study. J Investig Allergol Clin Immunol 2014;24(5):367–8.
80. Bircher AJ, Harr T, Hohenstein L, et al. Hypersensitivity reactions to anticoagulant drugs: diagnosis and management options. Allergy 2006;61(12):1432–40.
81. Bose S, Guyer A, Long A, et al. Evaluation and management of hypersensitivity to proton pump inhibitors. Ann Allergy Asthma Immunol 2013;111(6):452–7.
82. Bonadonna P, Lombardo C, Bortolami O, et al. Hypersensitivity to proton pump inhibitors: diagnostic accuracy of skin tests compared to oral provocation test. J Allergy Clin Immunol 2012;130(2):547–9.

Perioperative Anaphylaxis
Diagnosis, Evaluation, and Management

Jennifer A. Kannan, MD[a], Jonathan A. Bernstein, MD[a,b],*

KEYWORDS

- Anaphylaxis • Perioperative • Anesthesia • Asthma • Tryptase • NMBAs
- Antibiotics

KEY POINTS

- Perioperative anaphylaxis is becoming more common as the use of anesthesia and antibiotics increases. It can have fatal outcomes if not identified and treated quickly.
- Evaluation of a patient with a history of perioperative anaphylaxis requires a detailed medical history, a review of the anesthetic record, and collaboration between the anesthesiologist and the allergist.
- Testing to identify the implicated agents by skin testing, intracutaneous testing, and/or specific immunoglobulin E ideally should be performed 4 to 6 weeks after the event to ensure accuracy of the results.
- All asthmatic patients or patients with a remote history of asthma should ideally undergo a preoperative assessment of their lung function by spirometry and, if available, an exhaled nitric oxide test to assess their level of control.

INTRODUCTION

Anaphylaxis is defined as a serious, life-threatening generalized or systemic hypersensitivity reaction that is rapid in onset and may cause death.[1,2] Perioperative anaphylaxis can occur during surgery or postoperatively and present as cardiovascular collapse, airway obstruction, or arrest with or without skin manifestations.[3] Anaphylaxis has been classified into 4 grades depending on the severity of symptoms reported.[4] Grade I includes cutaneous signs, grade II includes non–life-threatening symptoms, grade III includes life-threatening symptoms such as arrhythmias and bronchospasm, and

Disclosure: The authors have nothing to disclose.
[a] Division of Immunology, Allergy and Rheumatology, Department of Medicine, University of Cincinnati College of Medicine, 3255 Eden Avenue, Suite 350, ML 563, Cincinnati, OH 45267-0563, USA; [b] Bernstein Clinical Research Center, 8444 Winton Road, Cincinnati, OH 45231, USA
* Corresponding author. Division of Immunology, Allergy and Rheumatology, University of Cincinnati, 3255 Eden Avenue, Suite 350, ML 563, Cincinnati, OH 45267-0563.
E-mail address: bernstja@ucmail.uc.edu

Immunol Allergy Clin N Am 35 (2015) 321–334
http://dx.doi.org/10.1016/j.iac.2015.01.002
0889-8561/15/$ – see front matter © 2015 Elsevier Inc. All rights reserved.

grade IV includes cardiac and respiratory distress.[4] Although its incidence is difficult to establish,[5] it is estimated to occur in 1 in 3500 to 1 in 20,000 surgeries, with a mortality ranging from 3% to 9 %.[4,6,7] Worldwide, it accounts for 9% to 19 % of all surgical complications and 5% to 7 % of all deaths during anesthesia.[6]

Anaphylaxis occurs as the result of a stimulus causing the release of bioactive mediators from mast cells and basophils in 2 or more organ systems of the body.[4,5] The release of mediators leads to extensive capillary permeability, vasodilation, bronchoconstriction, and hypotension associated with anaphylaxis.[4] When it occurs in relation to a drug, it is usually both unexpected and dose independent.[8,9] The mechanism may be immunoglobulin (Ig) E or non-IgE mediated, the latter including immune complex formation leading to activation of complement, or it can be related to direct histamine release.[1,6,7,10] Although most systemic anaphylaxis reactions are immediate, delayed reactions can occur.[4]

Perioperative anaphylaxis is becoming more common, most likely because of the increased frequency of using anesthesia and the increased complexity of anesthesia protocols.[3,7] Thus, it requires careful evaluation by the allergist in conjunction with the anesthesiologist to identify the cause so that safe anesthetic regimens can be recommended in the future.[3,4,6] This article presents 2 cases of perioperative anaphylaxis followed by a review of the approach for evaluating and managing patients who experience perioperative anaphylaxis and a discussion regarding the most commonly implicated agents.

Case 1

Patient 1 is a 72-year-old caucasian woman with a medical history of kidney stones, hypertension, diabetes mellitus, and hypothyroidism who presented after anaphylaxis during a cystoscopy. She had no prior history of asthma. She had undergone 3 lithotripsies and a knee surgery in the past without issues. Pertinent medications included atenolol 25 mg and diclofenac 75 mg once a day. On the day of her surgical procedure, she was given ciprofloxacin perioperatively, propofol, lidocaine, glycopyrrolate, and the anesthetic gases desflurane and sevoflurane intraoperatively. She also received Oxilan, a radiographic contrast media (RCM), during the procedure. In the recovery room, approximately 60 minutes after the conclusion of the procedure, the patient complained of chest tightness and then developed diffuse urticaria and hypotension. She was immediately treated with intramuscular (IM) epinephrine 0.03 mg 1:1000 and intravenous (IV) diphenhydramine 50 mg; a hand-held nebulizer treatment with albuterol and methylprednisolone 60 mg IV were also administered. Her hives rapidly resolved and her blood pressure normalized. Subsequent outpatient skin testing to lidocaine, propofol, glycopyrrolate, and ciprofloxacin was negative. This testing was followed by a challenge to each, which was negative as well. Based on her history it was presumed that the reaction was most likely secondary to the RCM. Recommendations were made to use low-osmolality contrast material and pretreat with corticosteroids and diphenhydramine according to published guidelines before any future procedures requiring RCM.[3,11]

Case 2

Patient 2 is a 24-year-old woman with a remote history of asthma not requiring treatment, allergic rhinitis, egg allergy, and atopic dermatitis who presented for further evaluation after 2 episodes of perioperative anaphylaxis. While undergoing anesthetic induction for the initial jaw surgery she developed hypotension, wheezing, and hypoxia leading to cardiopulmonary arrest. Surgery was immediately stopped and she was treated by anesthesia with epinephrine 0.3 mg 1:1000 IM, IV fluids, and IV corticosteroids. She was referred to an allergist and was subsequently tested to several medications that were administered perioperatively. She had positive intracutaneous skin testing to the neuromuscular blocking agents (NMBAs) vecuronium, succinylcholine, rocuronium, and cisatracurium. She was also skin test positive to penicillin, sulfamethoxazole, ciprofloxacin, and the first-generation cephalosporin cephalexin. These agents were all avoided during a second surgery; however, she again developed similar symptoms, including severe bronchospasm requiring epinephrine 0.3 mg 1:1000 IM, IV fluids, and corticosteroids. She was then referred to our clinic for further assessment. During her reevaluation, spirometry to assess asthma control revealed a forced expiratory volume in 1 second of 91% with 14% reversibility after bronchodilator and an exhaled nitric oxide level of 52 ppb. Serum tryptase, sedimentation rate, C-reactive protein, and thyroid-stimulating hormone were all normal. She was started on an inhaled corticosteroid, cetirizine 10 mg daily and a rescue short-acting beta-2 agonist, and an epinephrine injector was provided. Further review of the anesthetic record showed that before each surgery she was administered a β-blocker intraoperatively. It was thought that her uncontrolled asthma compounded with the use of a β-blocker resulted in respiratory arrest. Before her third surgery, after her asthma was deemed to be controlled, she was still empirically pretreated with prednisone and diphenhydramine to further mitigate the potential for any unforeseen complications. In addition, NMBAs and β-blockers were avoided. She was able to tolerate 2 subsequent surgeries successfully without complications.

EVALUATION

The manifestations of anaphylaxis during anesthesia can be different from anaphylaxis not associated with anesthesia, making the diagnosis of perioperative anaphylaxis more challenging.[7,12] For example, symptoms such as malaise, pruritus, dizziness, and dyspnea can be difficult to ascertain in an unconscious patient.[6,12] The most commonly reported objective features include pulselessness, ventilation difficulty, decreased end-tidal CO_2, and desaturation.[12] Other symptoms may include urticaria, flushing, skin rash, angioedema, nausea, vomiting, diarrhea, bronchospasm, rhinoconjunctivitis, and hypotension.[6,8] Although tachycardia can occur, bradycardia occurs more often, which can obfuscate the diagnosis.[3,6] The diagnosis may be even more difficult to determine in patients who are on preoperative β-blockers, which are frequently administered to reduce cardiovascular morbidity and mortality.[6,13]

Recognition of perioperative anaphylaxis is complicated, because patients are often sedated and therefore unable to alert physicians of symptoms. In addition, the diagnosis can be hampered because skin manifestations can be hidden by surgical drapes, cardiac events associated with anaphylaxis can be mistaken for other causes of cardiovascular collapse, and multiple drugs are frequently administered at the same time or in rapid succession.[3,6,12] Most of these reactions occur within minutes of administration of the suspected agent, but late-onset reactions can occur, depending on the agent and the timing of its administration.[6]

Treatment during the event should include cessation of the anesthetic or drug, rapid volume expansion, and prompt epinephrine administration.[2–5,14] Antihistamines are useful to treat skin manifestations and beta-adrenergic agonists should be used to treat bronchospasm.[6] Glucagon can be administered in patients on β-blockers or who have been administered a β-blocker perioperatively, to overcome epinephrine resistance.[2,3] Corticosteroids can be used for controlling the progression of bronchospasm and to prevent late-phase anaphylaxis.[4,6] The evaluation should begin with a thorough investigation of the anesthetic record regarding the details and timing of the event and medication administration (**Fig. 1**).[6,15] Medical history should include information regarding previous adverse drug reactions (**Fig. 2**).[3,4] All patients with a history of anaphylaxis during the perioperative period should have their medication list carefully reviewed for drugs that may place them at increased risk for anaphylaxis before any future surgeries.

RISK FACTORS

There are multiple risk factors associated with perioperative anaphylaxis that must be considered (**Fig. 3**). These risk factors include atopy; a previous history of reactions to anesthetic agents or other medications or products used during the procedure; multiple surgeries; latex allergy; children with spina bifida who have had multiple surgical interventions; allergic reactions to foods such as avocado, kiwi, banana, pineapple, papaya, chestnut, buckwheat, or *Ficus benjamina* that may cross react with latex[4,15,16]; systemic mastocytosis; and hereditary angioedema.[6]

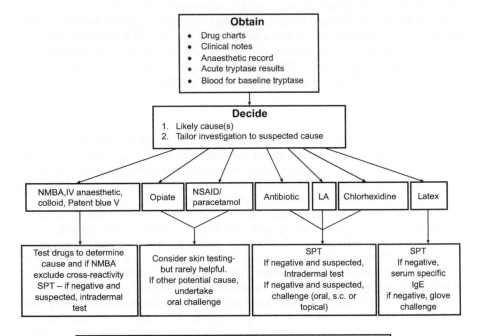

Fig. 1. Perioperative anaphylaxis evaluation. GP, general practitioner; NSAID, nonsteroidal antiinflammatory drug; s.c., subcutaneous; SPT, skin prick testing; LA, local anesthetics; MHRA, medicines and medical devices regulation. (*From* Ewan PW, Dugué P, Mirakian R, et al. BSACI guidelines for the investigation of suspected anaphylaxis during general anaesthesia. Clin Exp Allergy 2010;40(1):20; with permission.)

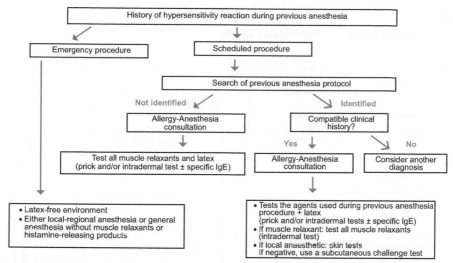

Fig. 2. Evaluation of a patient who has experienced a prior adverse reaction to anesthesia. (*From* Mertes PM, Malinovsky JM, Jouffroy L, et al. Working Group of the SFAR and SFA. Reducing the risk of anaphylaxis during anesthesia: 2011 updated guidelines for clinical practice. J Investig Allergol Clin Immunol 2011;21(6):450; with permission.)

Asthma, and especially uncontrolled asthma, is a known risk factor for all types of anaphylaxis because it is frequently a target organ.[17,18] Although volatile anesthetics have been shown in some studies to have a bronchodilatory effect and have been used in treatment of status asthmaticus,[19] bronchial hyperactivity and bronchospasm can occur at any point after administration of anesthesia during surgery.[17,18] This risk is increased if the asthma is uncontrolled, as shown by a recent asthma attack,[8] overuse of bronchodilators, or recent hospitalization for asthma.[20] Therefore, assessment of an asthma patient's level of control, which should include either spirometry or pulmonary function tests, is of paramount importance in the preoperative evaluation.[18,20] Patients with uncontrolled disease should be placed on inhaled corticosteroids and, if needed, a beta-2 agonist, because these have been shown to decrease bronchial hyperactivity during anesthesia.[4,6,18] With the exception of urgent or emergent indications, patients with uncontrolled asthma should have surgery postponed until optimal control is achieved. This important point is made in the case described earlier.

Patients with perioperative anaphylaxis should be queried for other rare systemic conditions that can predispose to anaphylaxis, such as hereditary angioedema[21–23] and systemic mastocytosis.[24,25] Atopic individuals may be at increased risk for more frequent and severe reactions.[3,26] These reactions are more common in women than in men, in particular with latex and NMBAs.[26] Although it is unclear whether β-blockers increase the risk of anaphylaxis, they can make it more difficult to treat these reactions.[3,4] Patients on this class of medication should be monitored closely. The above cases highlights the importance of these risk factors.

COMMONLY IMPLICATED AGENTS
Neuromuscular Blocking Agents

NMBAs are the most common cause of perioperative anaphylaxis, accounting for up to 60 to 70% of reported cases.[3,4,26–30] Rocuronium and succinylcholine are the most commonly implicated agents.[7] Anaphylaxis may occur either secondary to an

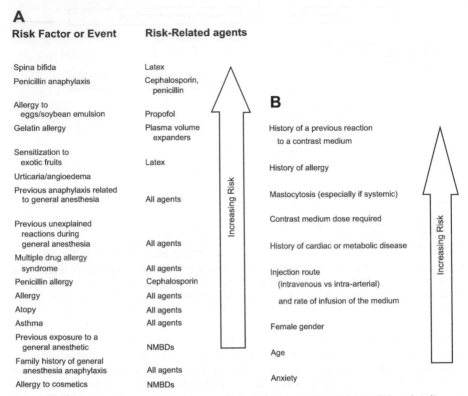

Fig. 3. Risk factors for increased risk of anaphylaxis for general anesthetics (*A*) and radiocontrast (*B*). (*From* Liccardi G, Lobefalo G, Di Florio E, et al, Hospital Radiocontrast Media and Anesthetic-Induced Anaphylaxis Prevention Working Group. Strategies for the prevention of asthmatic, anaphylactic and anaphylactoid reactions during the administration of anesthetics and/or contrast media. J Investig Allergol Clin Immunol 2008;18:3; with permission.)

IgE-mediated mechanism or from direct histamine release from mast cells.[3,6] Specific IgE sensitization is directed toward the tertiary or quaternary ammonium groups of these agents and is responsible for cross reactivity between NMBAs.[3,4,6,26] This cross reactivity occurs most commonly between vecuronium and pancuronium.[3] Other potential agents that cross react with NMBAs include choline, acetylcholine, morphine, neostigmine, and pentolium.[3] Pholcodine, an over-the-counter antitussive agent available in other countries, has also been reported to cross react with NMBAs.[31,32] Reactions are more common in women, and it is thought that cross reactivity of specific IgE with NMBAs can occur with the ammonium compound found in personal care products.[3,26]

Latex

Latex was the second most common agent responsible for perioperative anaphylaxis but the incidence has significantly decreased because most hospitals and outpatient surgical facilities have adopted latex-free policies.[4,6,26] Reactions tend to occur during the maintenance phase of anesthesia.[6] Children with a history of multiple surgeries, including those with spina bifida, spinal cord trauma, and urogenital malformations, were found to be of greatest risk for an IgE-mediated reaction to latex, with different epitopes of Hev b proteins being implicated.[26,33,34] In addition, patients with a history of allergy to specific foods that cross react with latex were found to be at increased risk, possibly related to lipid transfer proteins.[26,35] One case report describes a patient with latex sensitization and peach allergy who developed anaphylaxis during surgery, which highlights this important point.[36] Patients with a history of asthma and health care workers were also found to be at increased risk for latex anaphylaxis.[6,26]

Antibiotics

Antibiotics are frequently implicated in perioperative anaphylaxis.[3,27] These medications are commonly administered before and during surgery and reactions can be IgE or non-IgE mediated.[3] The most commonly associated antibiotics include β-lactams and vancomycin.[3] The highest cross reactivity exists with penicillins and first-generation cephalosporins; these reactions are becoming more common because of the increased use of perioperative antibiotic prophylaxis.[3,27] Although IgE-mediated anaphylaxis to vancomycin has been reported, reactions to this drug are more commonly non-IgE mediated, caused by direct histamine release resulting in red man syndrome, which is related to the infusion rate, with higher rates increasing the likelihood of histamine release.[3,6] IgE-mediated reactions to quinolones, rifampin, and bacitracin have also been reported.[17,37–40] Guidelines recommend that infusion of antibiotics occur while the patient is awake in order to better assess any reaction that develops.[4]

Hypnotics

Several cases of anaphylaxis to barbiturates, in particular thiopental, have been reported.[3,41,42] Specific IgE antibody reactions and direct histamine release have been implicated as mechanisms of action.[3,43] These reactions are most common in women.[3,44] Reactions to etomidate and ketamine are rare.[26,30,45] Atopy has been suggested to be a predisposing factor for nonspecific histamine release after ketamine.[26]

Propofol has been reported to cause IgE-mediated reactions with its 2 isopropyl groups acting as antigenic epitopes; however, most reactions are nonimmunologic secondary to direct histamine release.[3,6] This effect may be greater in the presence of NMBAs.[3] Although it has been proposed that patients allergic to egg and soy have an increased risk of anaphylaxis to propofol, there is no evidence to support this theory.[27]

Allergic reactions to IV diazepam are often caused by the propylene glycol solvent, which is sensitizing and can be found in medications, cosmetics, vaccines, and foods.[26,46] An IgE-mediated reaction to its metabolite has been proposed to be responsible for its cross reactivity with other benzodiazepines.[26]

Opioids

Anaphylaxis to narcotics in the perioperative period is rare and most commonly occurs through non–IgE-mediated nonspecific histamine release.[3,6,8,26,47] Most of the reactions include flushing, urticaria, pruritus, and mild hypotension.[3,8] Although fentanyl has not been shown to stimulate histamine release,[3,6,26] there are reports of IgE-mediated anaphylaxis to both morphine and fentanyl.[3,48–50] Reducing the rate of opioid administration limits the severity of these non–IgE-mediated reactions.[3]

Colloids

Colloids, or plasma volume expanders, include gelatin, albumin, hydroxyethyl starch (HES), and dextrans.[26,51,52] They are responsible for approximately 4% of all perioperative anaphylaxis cases.[26,53] Reactions to these agents are most common in men and in patients with a history of multiple drug allergies. Dextran and HES reactions are rare, occurring in less than 1% of all reactions.[3,54–56] Although specific IgG antibodies can be detected, their clinical significance is unknown.[3,52,57–60] Specific IgE antibodies have been detected to gelatin.[52,61] Gelatin is contained in many products, including foods, vaccines, pharmaceuticals, and cosmetics, and therefore exposure is common.[26,62] Case reports have described systemic reactions to albumin but it is unclear whether the mechanism is IgE or non-IgE mediated.[3,51,63]

Hemostatics

Intravenous protamine has been reported to cause anaphylactic reactions and IgG and IgE antibodies to protamine have been identified.[3,64] Case reports have proposed that they cross react with fish.[65] Anaphylaxis to aprotinin and thrombin has been reported along with detection of specific IgG and IgE antibodies.[66,67] Reactions to fibrin sealants have also been reported.[68]

Chlorhexidine

Chlorhexidine is a widely used antiseptic with the potential to cause various reactions, including irritant or allergic contact dermatitis, urticaria, and anaphylaxis.[6,8,69] Chlorhexidine is frequently used in the health care setting for its disinfectant properties but is also found in medical equipment, toothpaste, mouthwash, and household cleaning products.[69,70] Chlorhexidine IgE-mediated sensitization may occur through cutaneous, percutaneous, mucosal, and parenteral exposure.[69,70] It has been suggested that patients with a history of allergic contact dermatitis secondary to chlorhexidine may be at increased risk for anaphylaxis.[26] The incidence of reactions to chlorhexidine is thought to be underestimated.[8]

Blue Dyes

Blue dyes are commonly used intraoperatively for lymph node biopsy and sentinel lymph node dissection.[71,72] Blue dyes have been reported to rarely cause anaphylactic reactions, with the estimated incidence being 1% to 2%, with severe reactions compromising only 0.2% to 1.1% of cases.[7,71,72] Although cross-linkage of IgE antibodies and direct mast cell activation have been postulated,[72] reactions are more likely to occur secondary to the blue dye acting as a hapten binding to an endogenous protein forming a circulating complex capable of eliciting IgE sensitization.[71] It has been proposed that reactions secondary to blue dyes commonly develop as a result of their chemical similarity to isosulfan blue, a member of the triphenylmethane-based dye family commonly found in products such as cosmetics, soaps, antifungals, and paper industry materials.[26,71]

Nonsteroidal Antiinflammatory Drugs

Nonsteroidal antiinflammatory drugs (NSAIDs) inhibit cyclooxygenase, leading to the overproduction of leukotrienes.[8,26] These agents can produce bronchospasm, urticaria, and angioedema.[8] The mechanism for NSAID-induced anaphylaxis is most commonly non-IgE medicated but IgE-mediated reactions have been reported.[3,8,73] It has been reported that a prior reaction to a cyclooxygenase (COX) 1 inhibitor is a risk factor for subsequent reactions to a COX2 inhibitor.[26] However, this is inconclusive because patients who have experienced reactions to COX1 agents can often tolerate COX2 agents.[26] In one study, NSAIDs were the most common cause of anaphylaxis and were associated with a higher rate of repeat reactions.[74]

Other Agents

Angiotensin-converting enzyme inhibitors have been associated with non–IgE-mediated anaphylaxis.[73] Reactions to local anesthetics are uncommon and, when confirmed, reactions are more commonly found with ester versus amide agents.[3,75] One study found that 97% of skin tests to local anesthetics performed on patients with suspected local anesthetic allergy were negative.[76] Both immediate and delayed reactions have been reported to RCM, including anaphylaxis.[77,78] Risk factors for an RCM reaction include previous reaction to RCM, a history of cardiac disease, asthma, chronic kidney disease, β-blocker use, food allergy, drug allergy, contact allergy, and therapy with the cytokine interleukin-2.[26] However, neither seafood allergy nor allergy to iodine are risk factors for an RCM reaction.[27]

EVALUATION AND MANAGEMENT

Tryptase is a protease released from mast cells during immediate hypersensitivity reactions.[6] An increased tryptase level of more than 25 μg/L one to six hours after suspected anaphylaxis suggests mast cell activation and mediator release and supports the diagnosis.[3,4,24] However, a normal tryptase level does not rule out anaphylaxis.[3,6,24] A high tryptase level should be repeated a few days after the event to rule out other diseases associated with a persistently high tryptase level.[1,6,24] Additional diagnostic testing based on the patient's past history and the medications they were exposed to perioperatively is often warranted in order to determine the cause of the acute increase in tryptase level.[3] A plasma histamine level, if checked within minutes, may be helpful to indicate an anaphylactic reaction specifically involving basophils.[4] The value of urinary leukotrienes as a diagnostic marker has not been determined and total IgE levels have no diagnostic value.[4]

Patients who present with perioperative anaphylaxis should be evaluated by an allergist in close proximity to the reaction in order to identify the inciting agent to prevent reexposure and potentially fatal outcomes.[6] To begin, the allergist should request all intraoperative and postoperative records, including medication records and vital signs from the medical facility where the surgery was conducted if these are not available through an electronic medical record. Skin or serologic testing to the suspected agent should be deferred, ideally for 4 to 6 weeks after the reaction, to ensure that mast cells and basophils, respectively, are not refractory to activation.[3,4] Agents for testing can be obtained with advanced notice from the hospital pharmacy if the patient is in the inpatient setting, or with the help of the anesthesiologist who has access to many of these medications if the patient is being evaluated in the outpatient setting. If there is difficulty obtaining certain medications for testing, it is advisable to refer the patient to an academic center where these agents can be obtained more readily. Percutaneous followed by intracutaneous testing should be performed.[3,4,28] Because standardized agents are not available for most of these medications, it is important to perform skin testing using nonirritating concentrations in order to avoid false-positive reactions.[9,79] Mertes and colleagues[4] published guidelines with nonirritating concentrations of commonly used NMBAs, hypnotics, opioids, local anesthetics, chlorhexidine, and methylene blue. Nonirritating concentrations for some antibiotics have also been published.[80] When testing for agents with cross-reactive epitopes[27] such as local anesthetics, several different agents should be tested.[3,4] It is important to emphasize that skin testing is to detect IgE antibody and does not identify reactions elicited through nonimmunologic reactions.[3] Furthermore, intracutaneous testing can be falsely positive if too high a concentration is tested, causing an irritant reaction. If possible, titration testing in normal control subjects to identify the threshold concentration causing an irritant-induced response is ideal but this requires institutional review board approval.[4] Skin testing beginning with very low dilutions of suspected agents, ideally preservative free, should be performed in patients with a highly convincing history of anaphylaxis.[3] Skin testing has been shown to be valuable in evaluating anaphylaxis secondary to barbiturates, streptokinase, penicillin, insulin, local anesthetics, and latex.[3,26] In vitro testing for specific IgE antibodies has been reported for the quaternary ammonium group of muscle relaxants, thiopental, morphine, propofol, and latex.[3,4] Skin testing is not recommended for preanesthetic screening of subjects without a history of suspected reactions.[3]

Prevention of anaphylaxis should begin with review of the patient's previous medical records for any history of previous reaction.[6] In those with latex sensitization, a latex-free operating room should be arranged.[4,6] Both H1 and H2 antagonists in conjunction with corticosteroids are the most commonly used medications to treat anaphylaxis, although they do not always prevent the progression of a reaction.[4,81] Manfredi and colleagues[81] proposed a global anaphylactic risk score to identify patients who are at increased risk for anaphylaxis and who may benefit from a premedication protocol. Using a scale of calculated risk factors, it places patients into 3 categories of risk and suggests premedication protocols. However, this scale has yet to be validated in large populations. Preoperative corticosteroids may also be beneficial for patients with asthma to prevent asthma-related morbidity.[20] Increased use of electronic databases has also been useful for increasing the knowledge gap on appropriate treatment and monitoring of patients with previous perioperative anaphylactic reactions.[82]

SUMMARY

Perioperative anaphylaxis is becoming more common and thus recognition and evaluation by anesthesiologists in concert with allergists is of paramount importance.[3,4,7] Reactions require a careful evaluation of the medical and anesthetic record[4]; skin prick and, if appropriate, intracutaneous testing to suspected agents, should be performed 4 to 6 weeks after the event.[3,4] Risk factors, such as a history of a previous reaction to the inciting agents, a history of latex allergy, a history of ingested medications known to cause anaphylaxis, atopy, and asthma, should be considered before undergoing anesthesia.[3,4,6,15,18] As shown in the two cases discussed earlier, assessment of patients' asthma control is extremely important because failure to do so can have serious consequences.[4,6,18,20]

REFERENCES

1. Simons FE, Ardusso LR, Dimov V, et al. World allergy organization anaphylaxis guidelines: 2013 update of the evidence base. Int Arch Allergy Immunol 2013; 162:193–204.
2. Sampson HA, Munoz-Furlong A, Campbell RL, et al. Second symposium on the definition and management of anaphylaxis: summary report–Second National Institute of Allergy and Infectious Disease/Food Allergy and Anaphylaxis Network symposium. J Allergy Clin Immunol 2006;117:391–7.
3. Lieberman P, Nicklas RA, Oppenheimer J, et al. The diagnosis and management of anaphylaxis practice parameter: 2010 update. J Allergy Clin Immunol 2010; 126:477–80.e1–42.
4. Mertes PM, Malinovsky JM, Jouffroy L, et al. Reducing the risk of anaphylaxis during anesthesia: 2011 updated guidelines for clinical practice. J Investig Allergol Clin Immunol 2011;21:442–53.

5. Lagopoulos V, Gigi E. Anaphylactic and anaphylactoid reactions during the perioperative period. Hippokratia 2011;15:138–40.
6. Galvao VR, Giavina-Bianchi P, Castells M. Perioperative anaphylaxis. Curr Allergy Asthma Rep 2014;14:452.
7. Caimmi S, Caimmi D, Bernardini R, et al. Perioperative anaphylaxis: epidemiology. Int J Immunopathol Pharmacol 2011;24:S21–6.
8. Peroni DG, Sansotta N, Bernardini R, et al. Perioperative allergy: clinical manifestations. Int J Immunopathol Pharmacol 2011;24:S69–74.
9. Rive CM, Bourke J, Phillips EJ. Testing for drug hypersensitivity syndromes. Clin Biochem Rev 2013;34:15–38.
10. Johansson SG, Bieber T, Dahl R, et al. Revised nomenclature for allergy for global use: report of the Nomenclature Review Committee of the World Allergy Organization, 2003. J Allergy Clin Immunol 2004;113:832–6.
11. Greenberger PA, Patterson R, Kelly J, et al. Administration of radiographic contrast medial in high-risk patients. Invest Radiol 1980;15(6 Suppl):S40–3.
12. Mertes PM, Tajima K, Regnier-Kimmoun MA, et al. Perioperative anaphylaxis. Med Clin North Am 2010;94:761–89, xi.
13. Blessberger H, Kammler J, Domanovits H, et al. Perioperative beta-blockers for preventing surgery-related mortality and morbidity. Cochrane Database Syst Rev 2014;(9):CD004476.
14. Doherty GM, Chisakuta A, Crean P, et al. Anesthesia and the child with asthma. Paediatr Anaesth 2005;15:446–54.
15. Dewachter P, Mouton-Faivre C, Emala CW. Anaphylaxis and anesthesia: controversies and new insights. Anesthesiology 2009;111:1141–50.
16. Kim KT, Hussain H. Prevalence of food allergy in 137 latex-allergic patients. Allergy Asthma Proc 1999;20:95–7.
17. Michavila Gomez AV, Belver Gonzalez MT, Alvarez NC, et al. Perioperative anaphylactic reactions: review and procedure protocol in paediatrics. Allergol Immunopathol (Madr) 2013. [Epub ahead of print].
18. Liccardi G, Lobefalo G, Di Florio E, et al. Strategies for the prevention of asthmatic, anaphylactic and anaphylactoid reactions during the administration of anesthetics and/or contrast media. J Investig Allergol Clin Immunol 2008; 18:1–11.
19. Burburan SM, Xisto DG, Rocco PR. Anaesthetic management in asthma. Minerva Anestesiol 2007;73:357–65.
20. Tirumalasetty J, Grammer LC. Asthma, surgery, and general anesthesia: a review. J Asthma 2006;43:251–4.
21. Zuraw BL, Bernstein JA, Lang DM, et al. A focused parameter update: hereditary angioedema, acquired C1 inhibitor deficiency, and angiotensin-converting enzyme inhibitor-associated angioedema. J Allergy Clin Immunol 2013;131: 1491–3.
22. Bowen T, Cicardi M, Farkas H, et al. 2010 International consensus algorithm for the diagnosis, therapy and management of hereditary angioedema. Allergy Asthma Clin Immunol 2010;6:24.
23. Barbara DW, Ronan KP, Maddox DE, et al. Perioperative angioedema: background, diagnosis, and management. J Clin Anesth 2013;25:335–43.
24. Michalska-Krzanowska G. Tryptase in diagnosing adverse suspected anaphylactic reaction. Adv Clin Exp Med 2012;21:403–8.
25. Bridgman DE, Clarke R, Sadleir PH, et al. Systemic mastocytosis presenting as intraoperative anaphylaxis with atypical features: a report of two cases. Anaesth Intensive Care 2013;41:116–21.

26. Caffarelli C, Stringari G, Pajno GB, et al. Perioperative allergy: risk factors. Int J Immunopathol Pharmacol 2011;24:S27–34.

27. Dewachter P, Mouton-Faivre C, Castells MC, et al. Anesthesia in the patient with multiple drug allergies: are all allergies the same? Curr Opin Anaesthesiol 2011; 24:320–5.

28. Tamayo E, Rodriguez-Ceron G, Gomez-Herreras JI, et al. Prick-test evaluation to anaesthetics in patients attending a general allergy clinic. Eur J Anaesthesiol 2006;23:1031–6.

29. Dong SW, Mertes PM, Petitpain N, et al. Hypersensitivity reactions during anesthesia. Results from the ninth French survey (2005–2007). Minerva Anestesiol 2012;78:868–78.

30. Karila C, Brunet-Langot D, Labbez F, et al. Anaphylaxis during anesthesia: results of a 12-year survey at a French pediatric center. Allergy 2005;60:828–34.

31. Brusch AM, Clarke RC, Platt PR, et al. Exploring the link between pholcodine exposure and neuromuscular blocking agent anaphylaxis. Br J Clin Pharmacol 2014;78:14–23.

32. Johansson SG, Florvaag E, Oman H, et al. National pholcodine consumption and prevalence of IgE-sensitization: a multicentre study. Allergy 2010;65:498–502.

33. Slater JE, Vedvick T, Arthur-Smith A, et al. Identification, cloning, and sequence of a major allergen (Hev b 5) from natural rubber latex (*Hevea brasiliensis*). J Biol Chem 1996;271:25394–9.

34. Banerjee B, Kanitpong K, Fink JN, et al. Unique and shared IgE epitopes of Hev b 1 and Hev b 3 in latex allergy. Mol Immunol 2000;37:789–98.

35. Ebo DG, Hagendorens MM, Bridts CH, et al. Sensitization to cross-reactive carbohydrate determinants and the ubiquitous protein profilin: mimickers of allergy. Clin Exp Allergy 2004;34:137–44.

36. Lenchner KI, Ditto AM. A 62-year-old woman with 3 episodes of anaphylaxis. Ann Allergy Asthma Immunol 2005;95:14–8.

37. Aranda A, Mayorga C, Ariza A, et al. In vitro evaluation of IgE-mediated hypersensitivity reactions to quinolones. Allergy 2011;66:247–54.

38. Kim DH, Choi YH, Kim HS, et al. A case of serum sickness-like reaction and anaphylaxis - induced simultaneously by rifampin. Allergy Asthma Immunol Res 2014;6:183–5.

39. Fenniche S, Maalej S, Fekih L, et al. Manifestations of rifampicin-induced hypersensitivity. Presse Med 2003;32:1167–9 [in French].

40. Sharif S, Goldberg B. Detection of IgE antibodies to bacitracin using a commercially available streptavidin-linked solid phase in a patient with anaphylaxis to triple antibiotic ointment. Ann Allergy Asthma Immunol 2007;98:563–6.

41. Dolovich J, Evans S, Rosenbloom D, et al. Anaphylaxis due to thiopental sodium anesthesia. Can Med Assoc J 1980;123:292–4.

42. Chung DC. Anaphylaxis to thiopentone: a case report. Can Anaesth Soc J 1976; 23:319–22.

43. Harle DG, Baldo BA, Smal MA, et al. Detection of thiopentone-reactive IgE antibodies following anaphylactoid reactions during anaesthesia. Clin Allergy 1986; 16:493–8.

44. Birnbaum J, Porri F, Pradal M, et al. Allergy during anaesthesia. Clin Exp Allergy 1994;24:915–21.

45. Watkins J. Etomidate: an 'immunologically safe' anaesthetic agent. Anaesthesia 1983;38(Suppl):34–8.

46. Wilson KC, Reardon C, Farber HW. Propylene glycol toxicity in a patient receiving intravenous diazepam. N Engl J Med 2000;343:815.

47. Baldo BA, Pham NH. Histamine-releasing and allergenic properties of opioid analgesic drugs: resolving the two. Anaesth Intensive Care 2012;40:216–35.
48. Tomar GS, Tiwari AK, Chawla S, et al. Anaphylaxis related to fentanyl citrate. J Emerg Trauma Shock 2012;5:257–61.
49. Belso N, Kui R, Szegesdi I, et al. Propofol and fentanyl induced perioperative anaphylaxis. Br J Anaesth 2011;106:283–4.
50. Dewachter P, Lefebvre D, Kalaboka S, et al. An anaphylactic reaction to trans-dermal delivered fentanyl. Acta Anaesthesiol Scand 2009;53:1092–3.
51. Ring J, Messmer K. Incidence and severity of anaphylactoid reactions to colloid volume substitutes. Lancet 1977;1:466–9.
52. Ring J. Anaphylactoid reactions to intravenous solutions used for volume substi-tution. Clin Rev Allergy 1991;9:397–414.
53. Sakaguchi M, Kaneda H, Inouye S. A case of anaphylaxis to gelatin included in erythropoietin products. J Allergy Clin Immunol 1999;103:349–50.
54. Bothner U, Georgieff M, Vogt NH. Assessment of the safety and tolerance of 6% hydroxyethyl starch (200/0.5) solution: a randomized, controlled epidemiology study. Anesth Analg 1998;86:850–5.
55. Kim HJ, Kim SY, Oh MJ, et al. Anaphylaxis induced by hydroxyethyl starch during general anesthesia - a case report. Korean J Anesthesiol 2012;63:260–2.
56. Grundmann U, Heinzmann A, Schwering L, et al. Diagnostic approach identifying hydroxyethyl starch (HES) triggering a severe anaphylactic reaction during anesthesia in a 15-year-old boy. Klin Padiatr 2010;222:469–70.
57. Zinderman CE, Landow L, Wise RP. Anaphylactoid reactions to Dextran 40 and 70: reports to the United States Food and Drug Administration, 1969 to 2004. J Vasc Surg 2006;43:1004–9.
58. Hernandez D, de Rojas F, Martinez Escribano C, et al. Fatal dextran-induced allergic anaphylaxis. Allergy 2002;57:862.
59. Dieterich HJ, Kraft D, Sirtl C, et al. Hydroxyethyl starch antibodies in humans: incidence and clinical relevance. Anesth Analg 1998;86:1123–6.
60. Kreimeier U, Christ F, Kraft D, et al. Anaphylaxis due to hydroxyethyl-starch-reactive antibodies. Lancet 1995;346:49–50.
61. Luhmann SJ, Sucato DJ, Bacharier L, et al. Intraoperative anaphylaxis secondary to intraosseous gelatin administration. J Pediatr Orthop 2013;33:e58–60.
62. Khoriaty E, McClain CD, Permaul P, et al. Intraoperative anaphylaxis induced by the gelatin component of thrombin-soaked Gelfoam in a pediatric patient. Ann Allergy Asthma Immunol 2012;108:209–10.
63. Komericki P, Grims RH, Aberer W, et al. Near-fatal anaphylaxis caused by human serum albumin in fibrinogen and erythrocyte concentrates. Anaesthesia 2014;69:176–8.
64. Nyhan DP, Shampaine EL, Hirshman CA, et al. Single doses of intravenous prot-amine result in the formation of protamine-specific IgE and IgG antibodies. J Allergy Clin Immunol 1996;97:991–7.
65. Knape JT, Schuller JL, de Haan P, et al. An anaphylactic reaction to protamine in a patient allergic to fish. Anesthesiology 1981;55:324–5.
66. Prieto Garcia A, Villanueva A, Lain S, et al. Fatal intraoperative anaphylaxis after aprotinin administration. J Investig Allergol Clin Immunol 2008;18:136.
67. Wai Y, Tsui V, Peng Z, et al. Anaphylaxis from topical bovine thrombin (Thrombostat) during haemodialysis and evaluation of sensitization among a dial-ysis population. Clin Exp Allergy 2003;33:1730–4.
68. Schievink WI, Georganos SA, Maya MM, et al. Anaphylactic reactions to fibrin sealant injection for spontaneous spinal CSF leaks. Neurology 2008;70:885–7.

69. Toomey M. Preoperative chlorhexidine anaphylaxis in a patient scheduled for coronary artery bypass graft: a case report. AANA J 2013;81:209–14.
70. Opstrup MS, Malling HJ, Kroigaard M, et al. Standardized testing with chlorhexidine in perioperative allergy - a large single-centre evaluation. Allergy 2014; 69:1390–6.
71. Haque SH, Nossaman BD. Dyed but not dead. Ochsner J 2012;12:135–40.
72. Mertes PM, Malinovsky JM, Mouton-Faivre C, et al. Anaphylaxis to dyes during the perioperative period: reports of 14 clinical cases. J Allergy Clin Immunol 2008;122:348–52.
73. Jurakic Toncic R, Marinovic B, Lipozencic J. Nonallergic hypersensitivity to nonsteroidal antiinflammatory drugs, angiotensin-converting enzyme inhibitors, radiocontrast media, local anesthetics, volume substitutes and medications used in general anesthesia. Acta Dermatovenerol Croat 2009;17:54–69.
74. Faria E, Rodrigues-Cernadas J, Gaspar A, et al. Drug-induced anaphylaxis survey in Portuguese Allergy Departments. J Investig Allergol Clin Immunol 2014; 24:40–8.
75. Bhole MV, Manson AL, Seneviratne SL, et al. IgE-mediated allergy to local anaesthetics: separating fact from perception: a UK perspective. Br J Anaesth 2012; 108:903–11.
76. McClimon B, Rank M, Li J. The predictive value of skin testing in the diagnosis of local anesthetic allergy. Allergy Asthma Proc 2011;32:95–8.
77. Brockow K. Immediate and delayed reactions to radiocontrast media: is there an allergic mechanism? Immunol Allergy Clin North Am 2009;29:453–68.
78. Kim MH, Lee SY, Lee SE, et al. Anaphylaxis to iodinated contrast media: clinical characteristics related with development of anaphylactic shock. PLoS One 2014; 9:e100154.
79. Brockow K, Garvey LH, Aberer W, et al. Skin test concentrations for systemically administered drugs – an ENDA/EAACI Drug Allergy Interest Group position paper. Allergy 2013;68:702–12.
80. Broz P, Harr T, Hecking C, et al. Nonirritant intradermal skin test concentrations of ciprofloxacin, clarithromycin, and rifampicin. Allergy 2012;67:647–52.
81. Manfredi G, Pezzuto F, Balestrieri A, et al. Perioperative anaphylactic risk score for risk-oriented premedication. Transl Med UniSa 2013;7:12–7.
82. Freeman SG, Love NJ, Misbah SA, et al. Impact of national guidelines on reporting anaphylaxis during anaesthesia – an outcome audit. Acta Anaesthesiol Scand 2013;57:1287–92.

Anaphylaxis to Chemotherapy and Monoclonal Antibodies

Mariana C. Castells, MD, PhD

KEYWORDS

- Anaphylaxis • Chemotherapy • Platins • Taxenes • Rapid desensitization
- Monoclonal antibodies • Tryptase • Skin testing

KEY POINTS

- Drug-induced hypersensitivity reactions (HSRs) have increased in the last 10 years, compromising the safety of patients treated with chemotherapy and biologicals, including monoclonal antibodies (MoAbs).
- Skin testing can identify those with immunoglobulin (Ig)E-mediated HSRs.
- Tryptase, which is elevated in IgE-mediated and some non–IgE-mediated reactions, provides evidence of mast cell and/or basophil activation.
- The basophil activation test and specific soluble IgE are promising tools for diagnosis and identification of potentially sensitized patients.
- Rapid drug desensitization, a treatment modality aimed at preventing anaphylaxis, is available for patients with HSRs in need of first-line therapy.

INTRODUCTION

Drug-induced hypersensitivity reactions (HSRs) have increased in the last 10 years, compromising the safety of patients treated with chemotherapy and biologicals, including monoclonal antibodies (MoAbs).[1–3] Anaphylactic reactions induced by these agents have been underrecognized and underreported owing to the lack of definitive tests at the time of the reactions. Tryptase, a major mast cell protease, is elevated in the serum during anaphylactic reactions,[4] including reactions induced by chemotherapy and MoAbs, and its elevation correlates with the severity of the reactions; however, it is currently underutilized.[5] Retrospective skin testing is the most specific and sensitive in vivo test available to determine the culprit agent, but it is only available

The author has nothing to disclose.
Allergy Immunology Training Program, Drug Hypersensitivity and Desensitization Center, Mastocytosis Center, Brigham and Women's Hospital, Harvard Medical School, 1 Jimmy Fund Way, Boston, MA 02115, USA
E-mail address: mcastells@partners.org

for a minority of drugs, including[6,7] some MoAbs[8] and more recently for taxenes.[9] Because HSRs can be severe and even life threatening (such as anaphylaxis), the medication is avoided after a reaction and alternative medications used, many of which are considered second-line therapy. This switch can result in decreased life expectancy and decreased quality of life. Skin testing and risk stratification can define candidates for a new modality of retreatment for patients allergic to their first-line therapy, namely rapid drug desensitization (RDD).[10]

HSRs and anaphylaxis can occur with most chemotherapeutics and MoAbs and symptoms can be induced by IgE and non-IgE activation of mast cells and basophils.[11,12] Typically, symptoms include cutaneous manifestations, such as flushing and/or pruritus, which can progress to urticaria, angioedema, and full body erythema with or without symptoms of other organ involvement.[13] Respiratory symptoms such as cough, rhinitis, and dyspnea, and gastrointestinal symptoms such as abdominal pain and bloating, nausea, vomiting, and diarrhea can follow the initial cutaneous symptoms. In severe cases, these symptoms progress to hypotension and cardiovascular collapse and, without prompt use of intramuscular epinephrine, oxygen, and fluids, can lead to death within a few minutes. Atypical symptoms of hypersensitivity such as rigors and fever have been seen with MoAbs and oxaliplatin.[14] Reactions typically occur at the time of drug infusion, although some reactions are delayed by hours or days after exposure to the culprit medications and may herald acute and severe reactions on subsequent administration.[10] Predictors for hypersensitivity and anaphylaxis to chemotherapy and MoAbs are not available, but risk factors have been identified, such as multiple exposures[15] and BRCA mutations for patients treated with platins.[16]

HYPERSENSITIVITY AND ANAPHYLAXIS TO CHEMOTHERAPY DRUGS

The chemotherapy drugs most commonly involved in HSRs and anaphylaxis include platins, taxenes, doxorubicin, asparginase, and epipodophyllotoxins. The most typical manifestations include cutaneous, cardiovascular, gastrointestinal, and respiratory symptoms. Atypical manifestations of HSRs are seen with taxenes and oxaliplatin, and include hypertension, back and chest pain, and rigors.

Platins

In a growing variety of cancers, platins are being used for prolonged treatments aimed at inducing either a cure or a prolonged remission, and with this a significant increase in HSRs has occurred over the last decade. Although platins are small molecules that cannot elicit an immunologic response unless haptenized, jewelry workers exposed to platin salts can become sensitized through inhalation and develop asthma upon multiple exposures.[17] Similarly in cancer patients, the single risk factor that predicts HSRs to platins is an increased number of exposures (Tables 1 and 2). HSRs to platins are typically induced by IgE sensitization after multiple exposures and result in symptoms derived from mast cell/basophil activation and mediator release. Once a patient is sensitized, anaphylaxis can be induced by minuscule amounts of medication.[18] The most commonly used platins include carboplatin, cisplatin, and oxaliplatin. Of these, carboplatin is the agent with the most reported HSRs in patients with ovarian cancer, with up to 27% of HSRs in patients receiving more than 7 cycles.[19] BRCA carriers are at greatest risk; up to 40% of BCRA+ ovarian cancer patients can be sensitized after 10 exposures.[16] Children with gliomas and other central nervous system, tumors are at risk for reactions and a high incidence of anaphylaxis has been reported after several exposures.[20]

Table 1		
Frequent presentations of hypersensitivity reactions to different agents		
Agents	**No. of Infusions Before First Reaction**	**Symptoms**
Platins	6–8	Urticaria, pruritus, flushing, respiratory, cardiovascular (hypotension)
Taxanes	0–1	Pruritus, flushing, pain (lumbar), cardiovascular (hypertension/hypotension)
Biological agents	0–1 or >5	Fever, chills, rash, pruritus, respiratory, cardiovascular (hyper/hypotension)

Adapted from Mezzano V, Giavina-Bianchi P, Picard M, et al. Drug desensitization in the management of hypersensitivity reactions to monoclonal antibodies and chemotherapy. BioDrugs 2014;28:133–44; and Caiado J, Picard M. Diagnostic tools for hypersensitivity to platinum drugs and taxanes: skin testing, specific IgE, and mast cell/basophil mediators. Curr Allergy Asthma Rep 2014;14:451.

Symptoms induced by carboplatin are classical for IgE-mediated anaphylactic reactions, with pruritus, hives, shortness of breath, nausea, vomiting, and hypotension.[19] Oxaliplatin reactions can occur in up to 63% of patients with gastrointestinal cancers after multiple exposures. Wong and colleagues[14] described 18 men and 30 women presenting with HSRs to oxaliplatin after 8 exposures: 33% had anaphylaxis and 59% had positive skin tests. Atypical reactions included thrombocytopenia, hemolytic anemia, neurologic symptoms, fever, and rigors. All patients were successfully treated with RDD.

Table 2		
Clinical features of immediate hypersensitivity reactions to platinum drugs and taxanes		
Clinical Features	**Platinum Drugs (n = 94)**	**Taxanes (n = 51)**
Cutaneous (flushing, pruritus, urticaria), %	99	86
Cardiovascular (%)		
Hypertension	11	24
Presyncope	17	25
Hypotension	11	2
Syncope	6	8
Respiratory (%)		
Dyspnea	30	33
Desaturation	10	27
Throat tightness (%)	19	22
Gastrointestinal (nausea/vomiting/diarrhea), %	26	16
Neuromuscular (%)		
Back pain	1	39
Chest pain	23	59
Abdominal pain	20	25

From Caiado J, Picard M. Diagnostic tools for hypersensitivity to platinum drugs and taxanes: skin testing, specific IgE, and mast cell/basophil mediators. Curr Allergy Asthma Rep 2014;14:451; with permission.

Taxenes

Taxenes such as paclitaxel and docetaxel are used widely for gynecologic, breast, and lung cancers and newer generations such as abraxene and cabacitaxel are used for other malignancies.[21] Reactions to taxenes occur upon first or second exposure, suggesting direct activation of mast cells or basophils as the mechanism, but raising the possibility of cross-reacting epitopes such that patients would be sensitized through exposure to environmental allergens before taxene exposure.[3,22] Paclitaxel is isolated from the bark of the North American Pacific yew tree (*Taxus brevifolia*) and docetaxel is derived from the bark of the European yew tree (*Taxus baccata*). However, paclitaxel is also found in small amounts in the bark of walnut trees and there is a report of a patient sensitized to walnuts who reacted on first exposure to paclitaxel, suggesting that sensitization had occurred through exposure to walnuts.[23] Paclitaxel is insoluble in water and its diluent Cremophor has been thought to be the culprit for HSRs because Cremophor can activate basophils directly.[24] However, patients reacting to paclitaxel have been switched to docetaxel and have continued to have HSRs indicating that Cremophor is not the culprit for the HSR because docetaxel is diluted in polysorbate 80.[25,26] Recently, reactions to Abraxene, an albumin compounded paclitaxel, have been reported indicating that nondiluent, taxene-specific antigens are responsible for some of the reactions.[27] Reactions to taxenes can include flushing and hypotension, but symptoms atypical for HSRs such as hypertension and back or chest pain can occur during anaphylactic reactions.[10] More than 40% of patients reacted to paclitaxel in early clinical studies and the addition of steroids and antihistamines has reduced the rate of reactions to less than 1%.[28] Because patients are heavily premedicated when exposed to taxenes, early signs of anaphylaxis may not be present, such as cutaneous symptoms, and an abrupt presentation of hypotension with back pain may be the initial sign of anaphylaxis.

Doxorubicin

Antracyclines (doxorubicin and liposomal doxorubicin) are commonly used for hematologic malignancies, breast cancer, and other solid tumors. Liposomal doxorubicin has permitted the use of higher doses of the drug with less toxicity, including neutropenia and cardiotoxicity. However, because liposomes activate complement there has been an increase in the rate of HSRs. The reactions occur at the first or second infusion and include cutaneous, respiratory, and cardiovascular symptoms.[29]

L-Asparaginase

L-Asparaginase is a bacterial enzyme used for the treatment of acute lymphoblastic leukemia. It is highly immunogenic and IgG and IgE Abs can be rapidly formed after few exposures.[3] IgG Abs can bind to L-asparaginase decreasing its bioavailability and inactivating its functions; IgE Abs can cause HSRs, which can range from local induration with erythema and edema to anaphylaxis. HSRs are less frequent with the use of a pegylated form with lower immunogenicity.[30] Another option, substitution of the *Escherichia coli* form in patients with HSRs to the *E Chrysanthemi* form has been successful, triggering very few reactions. RDDs have been done successfully for patients reactive to all formulations.[31,32]

Epipodophyllotoxins (Teniposide/Etoposide)

Teniposide is used for acute lymphoblastic leukemias and etoposide for testicular tumors, small cell lung cancer, and ovarian cancer. Because Cremophor and polysorbate 80 are the diluents for these drugs, HSRs have been attributed to the diluents and can be severe including hypotension and anaphylaxis. Slow infusion rates and pre-medications, like those used for taxenes, have reduced the rate of some mild to moderate reactions, but have not prevented anaphylaxis. RDD have been successfully done for these medications.[1,33]

Monoclonal Antibodies

MoAb therapy has changed dramatically the long-term outcomes of inflammatory connective tissue diseases and cancers. Reactions to MoAbs include infusion reactions resulting from cytokine release and/or immune complex generation. They occur with the first or second exposure, are more frequently seen with murine MoAbs,[34] and are characterized by rigors, fever, joint pain, and hypotension in severe cases. Currently, chimeric, humanized, and human MoAbs have been engineered. They have less immunogenic potential and the frequency of these reactions has decreased.[35] Other HSRs to MoAbs are more classical in presentation, including cutaneous symptoms such as itching, urticaria, and flushing; anaphylaxis may occur and is characterized by respiratory distress, laryngeal edema, bronchospasm, and gastrointestinal and cardiovascular involvement. In some cases, patients may display fever, chills, and myalgia.[36] These reactions can occur in patients with multiple exposures and an IgE mechanism can be demonstrated.[37] Mild to moderate reactions may respond to decreased infusion rates, H1-antihistamines, and corticosteroids, but severe reactions require epinephrine and reexposure is not recommended unless the medication is given through a DDR protocol.[38] Vultaggio and colleagues[39] analyzed reported infliximab-induced immediate infusion reactions and reported that the majority of severe reactions occurred within 15 minutes of the infusion; cutaneous and respiratory symptoms were the most common clinical features.

Delayed reactions to MoAbs usually occur within the first 2 weeks of treatment and are associated with arthralgia, myalgia, cutaneous rashes, fever, urticaria, and pruritus. The clinical presentation of delayed reactions may be consistent with a classic serum sickness–like syndrome, characterized by the production of antibody to foreign immunoglobulin with formation of antigen–antibody complexes.[40] Patchy lung infiltrates and necrotizing vasculitis may be present with inflammatory infiltrates and complement deposition involving small blood vessels.[41] It has been reported that about 2.5% of patients receiving infliximab infusion develop serum sickness–like reactions and similar reactions have been reported for other MoAbs as follows: abciximab given for acute coronary syndromes, trastuzumab for breast cancer, rituximab for lymphoma, omalizumab for asthma, and natalizumab for multiple sclerosis.[42–44]

Infusion of MoAbs can cause massive release of cytokines such as tumor necrosis factor-α, interferon-γ, and interleukin-6 by binding to FcγRs on various immune cells (monocytes, macrophages, cytotoxic T cells, and natural killer cells) and leading to their activation and/or lysis and subsequent cytokine release.[45] These reactions can range from a flulike syndrome to multiorgan failure and can be associated with anaphylaxis.[46] Clinical manifestations of cytokine release syndrome and hypersensitivity may overlap with symptoms of flushing, pruritus, fever, hypotension, dyspnea, and tachycardia, necessitating epinephrine, fluid resuscitation, oxygen, and steroids.[35]

Acute systemic reaction to biologicals can be caused by antidrug antibodies (ADA).[47] Patients who develop antibodies to MoAbs are more likely to present with immediate infusion-related reactions. ADAs can be IgG (IgG1) or IgE and reactions from these 2 types of antibodies may be indistinguishable clinically.[39] Increased infliximab IgG Abs correlate with immediate infusion reactions.[48] Although data are lacking in humans, it is possible that IgG ADAs can activate directly circulating basophils, through FcγRs, and indirectly activate tissue mast cells through complement activation.[49] Vultaggio and colleagues[50] identified the presence of serum infliximab-specific ADA Abs in reactive patients and further detected circulating rituximab-specific IgE in patients with more severe reactions.

Infusion reactions to infliximab occur within the first 10 infusions and IgE-mediated events can occur within the first 5 administrations, typically with reexposure after a period of interruption of treatment.[51] IgE-mediated reactions may occur as a first dose, as in the case of cetuximab-induced reactions, with preexisting cross-reacting IgE against alpha-gal present on the MoAb.[52] Patients sensitized to alpha-gal are at risk for anaphylaxis when treated with cetuximab. Polysorbate is an additive present in omalizumab, erythropoietin, darbepoietin, and docetaxel, and has been associated with anaphylactic-like reactions.

Infliximab and Other Tumor Necrosis Factor-α Blockers

Infliximab is a chimeric anti–tumor necrosis factor-α blocking drug used for inflammatory bowel diseases and for inflammatory arthritidies (rheumatoid arthritis, psoriatic arthritis, ankylosing spondylitis). Acute HSRs occur in 3% to 5% of treatments during infusion or immediately after infusion and for up to 24 hours later and can range from mild cutaneous symptoms to hypotension and anaphylaxis. Some of these reactions result from IgE sensitization, are mediated by mast cell/basophil degranulation, and are identified by positive skin tests.

Delayed reactions from 24 hours to 14 days after infusion are less frequent and can present as maculopapular rashes, arthralgias, fever, and generalized malaise as in serum sickness–like reactions. Treatment with steroids has been helpful.

Cross-reactivity among tumor necrosis factor-α blockers is rare and patients can typically be switched to another drug such as etanercept or adalimumab after reacting to infliximab.

Trastuzumab

Trastuzumab is a recombinant humanized MoAb that recognizes the human extracellular domain of the epidermal growth factor receptor (EGFR) receptor (HER-2) and is used in breast cancer with HER-2 overexpression. Severe HSRs, including anaphylaxis, have been reported in 0.25% of patients after several exposures and skin testing has identified an IgE-induced mechanism for these reactions. Slow infusion and premedication have not been helpful in sensitized patients and for those whom trastuzumab is first-line therapy, desensitization is recommended.

Rituximab

Rituximab is a chimeric murine/human MoAb directed against CD20 on malignant and normal B cells. Its use has been expanded from lymphomas to refractory connective tissue disorders such as rheumatoid arthritis and antineutrophil cytoplasmic antibody–positive vasculitis, immune thrombocytopenic purpura, and polymiositis, in which the production of autoreactive IgG and other Abs is thought to cause inflammation and tissue damage. Rituximab-induced HSRs range from cytokine release syndrome (typically in large burden lymphomas), which can present on first or second exposure with symptoms of chills, fever, generalized malaise, hypotension, and desaturation, to IgE-mediated reactions after 4 or more exposures. The former reactions can be severe with high tumor burdens and decrease in intensity as the disease is controlled and the tumor burden decreased. In contrast, with IgE-sensitized patients who typically present with pruritus, urticaria, chest tightness, nausea, vomiting, or diarrhea after several infusions, with continued treatment reactions can progress inducing hypotension and anaphylaxis. Some patients present with a mixture of symptoms of cytokine storm and IgE-mediated symptoms. Skin testing has been helpful to detect IgE sensitization and to identify candidates for desensitization. Patients with positive skin tests are candidates for desensitization and IgE-mediated symptoms are controlled using desensitization protocols. However fever, chills, and generalized malaise may require the use of morphine derivatives, cyclooxygenase-1 inhibitors, and, in some cases, steroids as premedications.

Cetuximab

Cetuximab is a chimeric mouse/human MoAb that has competitive inhibitory binding to EGFR and is used in tumors with overexpression of EGFR such as colorectal cancer, non–small cell lung cancer, and head and neck epidermoid cancers. HSRs occur in up to 24% of the patients and in 3% to 4% of cases, these reactions are anaphylactic. Reactions can occur at first exposure, as seen in patients sensitized to galactose-alpha 1, 3-galactose (alpha-gal) in a portion of the cetuximab molecule. Sensitization to this portion has been observed in the Southern United States, including Virginia, in which patients became sensitized to alpha-gal through tick bites and reacted to alpha-gal antigen in meat. Patients reacting to cetuximab have HSRs occurring during their infusion or shortly after the infusion, indicating that the epitopes are readily available. These patients have positive skin tests and have been desensitized successfully when cetuximab was preferred as first-line therapy.

Skin Testing for Chemotherapy and Monoclonal Antibodies

Standardized testing has not been established and different testing concentrations have been reported. The general recommendation is to wait at least 2 to 4 weeks after a reaction has occurred before testing, to ensure that the skin test is not falsely negative after anaphylaxis. The reported sensitivity carboplatin skin testing is 85.7% with an 8% to 8.5% false-negative rate.[5] Carboplatin intradermal skin testing at doses of 1 and 10 mg/mL are used, which is equivalent to the concentration at which the drug is infused. However, intradermal skin testing at 10 mg/mL may cause local skin necrosis. In a small study of patients who had not been exposed to carboplatin for longer than 6 months, the negative predictive value with the lower intradermal dose of less than 10 mg was 47%. Patil and colleagues found that, out of 23 patients who were found initially to be skin test negative, 52% converted to a positive skin test after exposure and 83% of these patients had additional HSRs, even with a desensitization protocol.[6,10]

Brennan and colleagues[8] reported skin test data on MoAbs, including skin prick and intradermal concentrations against rituximab, infliximab, and tratuzumab (**Table 3**). Vultaggio and colleagues found 7 positive skin tests out of 23 patients (30.4%) with infliximab allergy.[39] However, the patients with positive skin testing were more likely to have experienced a severe reaction defined as grade 3 anaphylaxis by the Brown criteria. Some drugs cannot be skin tested because of cutaneous toxicity, such as the vesicant agents, which can induce a blistering lesion at the site of skin testing (ie, liposomal doxorubicin, vincristine). Markman and colleagues[53] prospectively evaluated the predictive value of skin testing after 6 doses of carboplatin in 126 women with ovarian carcinoma and no history of HSRs during infusions. Of 87 skin test–negative women, 7 experienced an HSR during subsequent infusions, with a false-negative rate of 8%. Therefore, prophylactic skin testing for patients undergoing carboplatin treatment is not recommended.

Cross-reactive HSRs to cisplatin have been reported in as many as 30% of patients with a history of reactions to carboplatin.[54] Patients with a history of carboplatin reactions can be given cisplatin successfully if skin testing to cisplatin is negative.

Table 3
Skin testing doses for chemotherapeutic agents and monoclonal antibodies

Agent/Antibody	Skin Prick (mg/mL)	Intradermal (mg/mL)	Intradermal (mg/mL)	Intradermal (mg/mL)
Carboplatin	10	1	5–10	
Cisplatin	1	0.1	1	
Oxaliplatin	5	0.5	5	
Paclitaxel	1–6	0.001	0.01	
Abatacept (Castells et al, unpublished, 2014)	25	0.025	0.25	2.5
Etanercept (Castells et al, unpublished, 2014)	50	0.05	0.5	5
Infliximab	10	0.1	1	N/A
Rituximab	10	0.01	0.1	1
Trastuzumab	21	0.21	2.1	N/A

Abbreviation: N/A, not applicable.
Data from Wong JT, Ling M, Patil S, et al. Oxaliplatin hypersensitivity: evaluation, implications of skin testing, and desensitization. J Allergy Clin Immunol Pract 2014;2:40–5; and Brennan PJ, Rodriguez Bouza T, Hsu FI, et al. Hypersensitivity reactions to mAbs: 105 desensitizations in 23 patients, from evaluation to treatment. J Allergy Clin Immunol 2009;124:1259–66.

Caiado and colleagues[55] showed that in vitro testing may be used to identify platin-reacting patients. Carboplatin-specific IgE was found to be more specific, but less sensitive, whereas oxaliplatin-specific IgE had a higher sensitivity, but lower specificity. Patients sensitized to carboplatin may be able to tolerate oxaliplatin, but owing to its higher immunogenicity, patients sensitized to oxaliplatin may be at risk for an HSR if exposed to either carboplatin or cisplatin (**Table 4**). Madrigal-Burgaleta and associates[56] found oxaliplatin-specific IgE in 23 oxaliplatin-reactive patients, reporting a 38% sensitivity and 100% specificity in patients with mild to moderate reactions.

Basophils play important roles in allergic diseases through their release of inflammatory mediators. When specific allergens cross-link IgE bound to its high-affinity receptor, a basophil may express rapidly surface molecules such as CD203c and CD63, such as seen in the basophil activation test. Five patients who developed grade 2 to 4 anaphylaxis to carboplatin had high CD203c+ basophils, suggesting that basophil CD203c may be a promising biomarker in predicting carboplatin-induced anaphylaxis.[57]

Tryptase in Hypersensitivity Reactions and in Anaphylaxis to Chemotherapy and Monoclonal Antibodies

Tryptase is a protease present in all human mast cells and, in small amounts, in basophils. It is released from mast cell granules during allergic and anaphylactic reactions. Baseline elevation of serum tryptase is seen in patients with mastocytosis, renal failure, and chronic myeloid leukemia, but acute elevations are seen with anaphylaxis, including medication-induced anaphylaxis. IgE-mediated activation of mast cell and basophils triggers tryptase release within 30 to 60 minutes from the onset of symptoms tryptase concentrations correlate with severity of symptoms, with patients experiencing hypotension having higher serum tryptase values. Patients with HSR to chemotherapy including carboplatin have shown elevations of tryptase 5. Elevated tryptase has also been shown with non–IgE-mediated reactions (negative skin tests), such as those to taxanes and MoAbs. Tryptase measurement is important in determining the mechanism of HSRs, with elevated concentrations providing evidence of

Table 4
Carboplatin- and oxaliplatin-specific IgE: Cross-reactivity among carboplatin- and oxaliplatin-treated patients

Patient No.	Grade of the Initial Reaction	Skin Testing	Crb sIgE (kU_A/L)	Ox sIgE (kU_A/L)	Cis sIgE (kU_A/L)	Patient No.	Grade of the Initial Reaction	Skin Testing	Ox sIgE (kU_A/L)	Crb sIgE (kU_A/L)	Cis sIgE (kU_A/L)
		Crb-Sensitive Group						Ox-Sensitive Group			
1	3	0.1 ID	<0.10	<0.10	<0.10	13	2	5 SPT	0.16	1.60	0.68
2	3	10 SPT	<0.10	<0.10	<0.10	14	2	0.5 ID	2.80	1.70	1.95
3	2	1 ID	1.20	<0.10	0.72	15	1	0.5 ID	0.22	0.31	0.23
4	2	0.1 ID	<0.10	<0.10	<0.10	16	2	0.5 ID	4.9	8.8	10.6
5	3	0.1 ID	0.14	<0.10	<0.10	17	2	0.5 ID	1.5	<0.10	<0.10
6	3	1 ID	8.9	<0.10	<0.10	18	1	0.5 ID	<0.10	<0.10	<0.10
7	2	1 ID	1.2	<0.10	1.12	19	2	5 SPT	0.5	0.31	0.29
8	3	10 SPT	<0.10	<0.10	<0.10	20	2	ND	0.61	0.71	0.96
9	3	10 SPT	0.18	<0.10	<0.10	21	1	0.5 ID	<0.10	<0.10	<0.10
10	1	1 ID	<0.10	<0.10	ND	22	2	ND	0.61	0.63	0.67
11	3	10 SPT	0.85	<0.10	ND	23	3	0.5 ID	0.51	0.90	0.90
12	3	1 ID	0.49	<0.10	ND	24	1	0.5 ID	<0.10	<0.10	<0.10

Note. Bold values represent positive results.

Abbreviations: Cis, Cisplatin; Crb, carboplatin; ID, intradermal; IgE, immunoglobulin E; ND, not done; Ox, oxaliplatin; sIgE, specific IgE; SPT, skin prick test.

From Caiado J, Venemalm L, Pereira-Santos MC, et al. Carboplatin-, oxaliplatin-, and cisplatin-specific IgE: cross-reactivity and value in the diagnosis of carboplatin and oxaliplatin Allergy. J Allergy Clin Immunol Pract 2013;1:494–500; with permission.

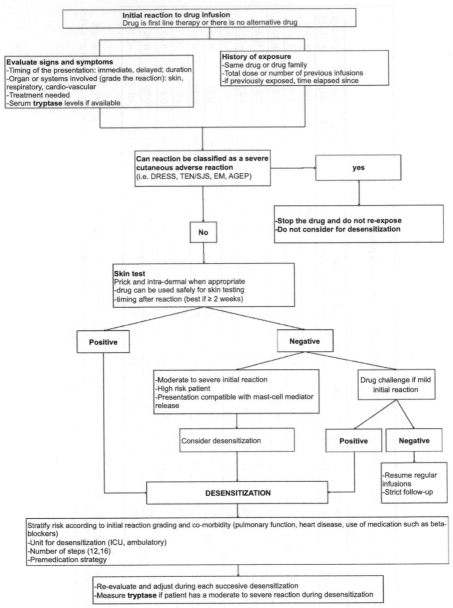

Fig. 1. Evaluation of drug hypersensitivity and anaphylaxis for chemotherapy and biologicals. AGE, acute generalized exanthematous pustulosis; DRESS, drug reaction with eosinophilia and systemic symptoms; EM, erythema multiforme; ICU, intensive care unit; SJS, Stevens–Johnson syndrome; TEN, toxic epidermal necrolysis. (*From* Mezzano V, Giavina-Bianchi P, Picard M, et al. Drug desensitization in the management of hypersensitivity reactions to monoclonal antibodies and chemotherapy. BioDrugs 2014;28:133–44; with permission).

mast cell/basophil activation and helping to determine the indication for desensitization if required. If tryptase is elevated at the time of the reaction, a second measurement at baseline is necessary to screen for mastocytosis.

Rapid Drug Desensitization for the Treatment of Anaphylaxis to Chemotherapy and Monoclonal Antibodies

In vitro desensitization of mast cells and basophils prevents the release of preformed mediators and inhibits cellular calcium entry, as well as the generation of prostaglandins, leukotrienes, and proinflammatory cytokines.[58,59] A mouse model of in vitro desensitization prevented anaphylaxis and death in sensitized animals when exposed to the sensitizing allergens.[60] Based on in vitro and in vivo data, desensitization protocols have been generated and used successfully in several hundred drug allergic patients (**Fig. 1**). These in vitro protocols can be used to determine the antigen dose eliciting a reaction based on the patient's circulating IgE level.

The Brigham and Women's Hospital/Dana Farber Cancer Institute desensitization program produced a 12-step standard protocol in which unresponsiveness to a triggering antigen dose was achieved by delivering doubling doses of antigen at fixed time intervals.[21] The protocol is based on 3 bags of medication administered sequentially starting with the bag containing a 1/100 dilution, then a 1/10 dilution and a full concentration of the chemotherapy agent to which the patient had an HSR (see **Table 3**). Patients who react to the protocol starting with the 1/100 dilution may start with a bag containing a 1/1000 dilution, with a 4-bag protocol. Patients need to be desensitized for each drug exposure and each desensitization protocol is customized to the specific dose so that patients receive the full therapeutic dose through the desensitization protocol.

SUMMARY

Anaphylaxis can occur with chemotherapy drugs. MoAbs and skin testing can identify those with IgE-mediated HSRs. Tryptase is elevated in IgE-mediated and some of the non–IgE-mediated reactions, and provides evidence of mast cell and/or basophil activation. Basophil activation test and specific soluble IgE are promising tools for the diagnosis and identification of potentially sensitized patients. For example, platin-exposed patients could be assessed for anti-platin IgE Abs after several exposures and, if positive, desensitization would be recommended, preventing anaphylactic reactions. RDD is a treatment modality aimed at preventing anaphylaxis and available for patients with HSRs in need of first-line therapy.

REFERENCES

1. Weiss RB. Hypersensitivity reactions. Semin Oncol 1992;19:458–77.
2. Sakaeda T, Kadoyama K, Yabuuchi H, et al. Platinum agent-induced hypersensitivity reactions: data mining of the public version of the FDA adverse event reporting system, AERS. Int J Med Sci 2011;8:332–8.
3. Kadoyama K, Kuwahara A, Yamamori M, et al. Hypersensitivity reactions to anti-cancer agents: data mining of the public version of the FDA adverse event reporting system, AERS. J Exp Clin Cancer Res 2011;30:93.
4. Schwartz LB. Diagnostic value of tryptase in anaphylaxis and mastocytosis. Immunol Allergy Clin N Am 2006;26:451–63.
5. Hesterberg PE, Banerji A, Oren E, et al. Risk stratification for desensitization of patients with carboplatin hypersensitivity: clinical presentation and management. J Allergy Clin Immunol 2009;123:1262–7.e1.

6. Patil SU, Long AA, Ling M, et al. A protocol for risk stratification of patients with carboplatin-induced hypersensitivity reactions. J Allergy Clin Immunol 2012; 129:443–7.

7. Lee CW, Matulonis UA, Castells MC. Carboplatin hypersensitivity: a 6-h 12-step protocol effective in 35 desensitizations in patients with gynecological malignancies and mast cell/IgE-mediated reactions. Gynecol Oncol 2004;95:370–6.

8. Brennan PJ, Rodriguez Bouza T, Hsu FI, et al. Hypersensitivity reactions to mAbs: 105 desensitizations in 23 patients, from evaluation to treatment. J Allergy Clin Immunol 2009;124:1259–66.

9. Prieto Garcia A, Pineda de la Losa F. Immunoglobulin E-mediated severe anaphylaxis to paclitaxel. J Investig Allergol Clin Immunol 2010;20:170–1.

10. Castells MC, Tennant NM, Sloane DE, et al. Hypersensitivity reactions to chemotherapy: outcomes and safety of rapid desensitization in 413 cases. J Allergy Clin Immunol 2008;122(3):574–80.

11. del Carmen Sancho M, Breslow R, Sloane D, et al. Desensitization for hypersensitivity reactions to medications. Chem Immunol Allergy 2012;97:217–33.

12. McNeil BD, Pundir P, Meeker S, et al. Identification of a mast-cell-specific receptor crucial for pseudo-allergic drug reactions. Nature 2014. [Epub ahead of print].

13. Hsu Blatman KS, Castells MC. Desensitizations for chemotherapy and monoclonal antibodies: indications and outcomes. Curr Allergy Asthma Rep 2014; 14:453.

14. Wong JT, Ling M, Patil S, et al. Oxaliplatin hypersensitivity: evaluation, implications of skin testing, and desensitization. J Allergy Clin Immunol Pract 2014;2:40–5.

15. Mezzano V, Giavina-Bianchi P, Picard M, et al. Drug desensitization in the management of hypersensitivity reactions to monoclonal antibodies and chemotherapy. BioDrugs 2014;28:133–44.

16. Moon DH, Lee JM, Noonan AM, et al. Deleterious BRCA1/2 mutation is an independent risk factor for carboplatin hypersensitivity reactions. Br J Cancer 2013; 109:1072–8.

17. Cristaudo A, Sera F, Severino V, et al. Occupational hypersensitivity to metal salts, including platinum, in the secondary industry. Allergy 2005;60:159–64.

18. Markman M, Kennedy A, Webster K, et al. Clinical features of hypersensitivity reactions to carboplatin. J Clin Oncol 1999;17:1141.

19. Navo M, Kunthur A, Badell ML, et al. Evaluation of the incidence of carboplatin hypersensitivity reactions in cancer patients. Gynecol Oncol 2006;103:608–13.

20. Lazzareschi I, Ruggiero A, Riccardi R, et al. Hypersensitivity reactions to carboplatin in children. J Neurooncol 2002;58:33–7.

21. Castells M. Desensitization for drug allergy. Curr Opin Allergy Clin Immunol 2006; 6:476–81.

22. Banerji A, Lax T, Guyer A, et al. Management of hypersensitivity reactions to Carboplatin and Paclitaxel in an outpatient oncology infusion center: a 5-year review. J Allergy Clin Immunol Pract 2014;2:428–33.

23. Feldweg AM, Lee CW, Matulonis UA, et al. Rapid desensitization for hypersensitivity reactions to paclitaxel and docetaxel: a new standard protocol used in 77 successful treatments. Gynecol Oncol 2005;96:824–9.

24. Decorti G, Bartoli Klugmann F, Candussio L, et al. Effect of paclitaxel and Cremophor EL on mast cell histamine secretion and their interaction with adriamycin. Anticancer Res 1996;16:317–20.

25. A fatal anaphylactic reaction to paclitaxel is described, which was preceded by a possible delayed reaction to the initial infusion. Allergy Asthma Proc 2011;32:79.

26. Denman JP, Gilbar PJ, Abdi EA. Hypersensitivity reaction (HSR) to docetaxel after a previous HSR to paclitaxel. J Clin Oncol 2002;20:2760–1.
27. Fader AN, Rose PG. Abraxane for the treatment of gynecologic cancer patients with severe hypersensitivity reactions to paclitaxel. Int J Gynecol Cancer 2009;19: 1281–3.
28. Huddleston R, Berkheimer C, Landis S, et al. Improving patient outcomes in an ambulatory infusion setting: decreasing infusion reactions of patients receiving paclitaxel and carboplatin. J Infus Nurs 2005;28:170–2.
29. Weiss RB, Bruno S. Hypersensitivity reactions to cancer chemotherapeutic agents. Ann Intern Med 1981;94:66–72.
30. Stone HD Jr, DiPiro C, Davis PC, et al. Hypersensitivity reactions to Escherichia coli-derived polyethylene glycolated-asparaginase associated with subsequent immediate skin test reactivity to E. coli-derived granulocyte colony-stimulating factor. J Allergy Clin Immunol 1998;101:429–31.
31. Soyer OU, Aytac S, Tuncer A, et al. Alternative algorithm for L-asparaginase allergy in children with acute lymphoblastic leukemia. J Allergy Clin Immunol 2009;123:895–9.
32. Guo Y. Desensitization therapy of acute lymphocytic leukemia with injection of L-asparaginase (Report of 5 cases). Zhonghua Er Ke Za Zhi 2005;43:309–10 [in Chinese].
33. O'Dwyer PJ, Weiss RB. Hypersensitivity reactions induced by etoposide. Cancer Treat Rep 1984;68:959–61.
34. Hong DI, Bankova L, Cahill KN, et al. Allergy to monoclonal antibodies: cutting-edge desensitization methods for cutting-edge therapies. Expert Rev Clin Immunol 2012;8:43–52 [quiz: 53–4].
35. Vultaggio A, Castells MC. Hypersensitivity reactions to biologic agents. Immunol Allergy Clin N Am 2014;34:615–32, ix.
36. Cheifetz A, Mayer L. Monoclonal antibodies, immunogenicity, and associated infusion reactions. Mt Sinai J Med 2005;72:250–6.
37. Cernadas JR, Brockow K, Romano A, et al. General considerations on rapid desensitization for drug hypersensitivity - a consensus statement. Allergy 2010; 65:1357–66.
38. Kang SP, Saif MW. Infusion-related and hypersensitivity reactions of monoclonal antibodies used to treat colorectal cancer-Identification, prevention, and management. J Support Oncol 2007;5:451–7.
39. Vultaggio A, Matucci A, Nencini F, et al. Anti-infliximab IgE and non-IgE antibodies and induction of infusion-related severe anaphylactic reactions. Allergy 2010;65:657–61.
40. Bavbek S, Ataman S, Bankova L, et al. Injection site reaction to adalimumab: positive skin test and successful rapid desensitisation. Allergol Immunopathol (Madr) 2013;41:204–6.
41. Dereure O, Navarro R, Rossi JF, et al. Rituximab-induced vasculitis. Dermatology 2001;203:83–4.
42. D'Arcy CA, Mannik M. Serum sickness secondary to treatment with the murine-human chimeric antibody IDEC-C2B8 (rituximab). Arthritis Rheum 2001;44: 1717–8.
43. Gamarra RM, McGraw SD, Drelichman VS, et al. Serum sickness-like reactions in patients receiving intravenous infliximab. J Emerg Med 2006;30:41–4.
44. Pilette C, Coppens N, Houssiau FA, et al. Severe serum sickness-like syndrome after omalizumab therapy for asthma. J Allergy Clin Immunol 2007; 120:972–3.

45. Stallmach A, Giese T, Schmidt C, et al. Severe anaphylactic reaction to infliximab: successful treatment with adalimumab - report of a case. Eur J Gastroenterol Hepatol 2004;16:627–30.
46. Castells M, Pichler WJ. Drug desensitization in oncology: chemotherapy agents and monoclonal antibodies. In: Pichler W, editor. Drug hypersensitivity. New York: Karger; 2007. p. 413–25.
47. Chung CH, Mirakhur B, Chan E, et al. Cetuximab-induced anaphylaxis and IgE specific for galactose-alpha-1,3-galactose. N Engl J Med 2008;358:1109–17.
48. Wolbink GJ, Vis M, Lems W, et al. Development of antiinfliximab antibodies and relationship to clinical response in patients with rheumatoid arthritis. Arthritis Rheum 2006;54:711–5.
49. Finkelman FD. Anaphylaxis: lessons from mouse models. J Allergy Clin Immunol 2007;120:506–15.
50. Vultaggio A, Matucci A, Nencini F, et al. Skin testing and infliximab-specific antibodies detection as a combined strategy for preventing infusion reaction. Intern Emerg Med 2012;7(Suppl 2):S77–9.
51. Jacobstein DA, Markowitz JE, Kirschner BS, et al. Premedication and infusion reactions with infliximab: results from a pediatric inflammatory bowel disease consortium. Inflamm Bowel Dis 2005;11:442–6.
52. Commins SP, Platts-Mills TA. Anaphylaxis syndromes related to a new mammalian cross-reactive carbohydrate determinant. J Allergy Clin Immunol 2009;124: 652–7.
53. Markman M, Zanotti K, Peterson G, et al. Expanded experience with an intradermal skin test to predict for the presence or absence of carboplatin hypersensitivity. J Clin Oncol 2003;21:4611–4.
54. Callahan MB, Lachance JA, Stone RL, et al. Use of cisplatin without desensitization after carboplatin hypersensitivity reaction in epithelial ovarian and primary peritoneal cancer. Am J Obstet Gynecol 2007;197:199.e1–4 [discussion: 199.e4–5].
55. Caiado J, Venemalm L, Pereira-Santos MC, et al. Carboplatin-, oxaliplatin-, and cisplatin-specific IgE: cross-reactivity and value in the diagnosis of carboplatin and oxaliplatin allergy. J Allergy Clin Immunol Pract 2013;1:494–500.
56. Madrigal-Burgaleta R, Berges-Gimeno MP, Angel-Pereira D, et al. Hypersensitivity and desensitization to antineoplastic agents: outcomes of 189 procedures with a new short protocol and novel diagnostic tools assessment. Allergy 2013;68: 853–61.
57. Iwamoto T, Yuta A, Tabata T, et al. Evaluation of basophil CD203c as a predictor of carboplatin-related hypersensitivity reaction in patients with gynecologic cancer. Biol Pharm Bull 2012;35:1487–95.
58. Morales AR, Shah N, Castells M. Antigen-IgE desensitization in signal transducer and activator of transcription 6-deficient mast cells by suboptimal doses of antigen. Ann Allergy Asthma Immunol 2005;94:575–80.
59. Zhao W, Gomez G, Macey M, et al. In vitro desensitization of human skin mast cells. J Clin Immunol 2012;32:150–60.
60. Oka T, Rios EJ, Tsai M, et al. Rapid desensitization induces internalization of antigen-specific IgE on mouse mast cells. J Allergy Clin Immunol 2013;132: 922–32.e1–16.

Idiopathic Anaphylaxis

Nana Fenny, MD, MPH, Leslie C. Grammer, MD*

KEYWORDS

• Anaphylaxis • Idiopathic anaphylaxis • Mast cell activation syndrome

KEY POINTS

• Idiopathic anaphylaxis (IA) is a diagnosis of exclusion after other causes, such as foods, medications, exercise, insect stings, C1 esterase inhibitor deficiency, and mastocytosis, have been excluded.

• A significant proportion (24%–59%) of anaphylaxis cases are classified as idiopathic in several reported patient series. There is a higher prevalence of idiopathic anaphylaxis in women compared with men and a high prevalence of atopy in patients with IA.

• Classification of IA is based on frequency of episodes and clinical manifestations; frequent episodes are defined as at least 2 episodes in the preceding 2 months or at least 6 episodes in the preceding year.

• Treatment of IA is individualized based on severity and frequency of symptoms.

• Acute treatment of IA is the same as treatment of anaphylaxis from other causes, except that prolonged tapering of prednisone is usually required to induce remission. All patients should possess an epinephrine autoinjector and an anaphylaxis emergency plan.

• The prognosis of IA is generally favorable with appropriate treatment and patient education.

BACKGROUND AND DEFINITION

The term idiopathic anaphylaxis (IA) refers to anaphylaxis without a discernible cause after completion of an appropriate diagnostic evaluation. It is a diagnosis of exclusion after other causes, such as foods, medications, exercise, insect stings, C1 esterase inhibitor deficiency, and mastocytosis, have been thoroughly considered and excluded. In 1978, Bacal and colleagues[1] reported the first cases of IA. In that report, of the 21 patients in the series, 11 had no causal explanation for anaphylaxis and the term IA was given. Initially, the medical community received the term IA with considerable doubt and skepticism because it was thought that an external cause or factors should

Supported by the Ernest S. Bazley Grant to Northwestern University and Northwestern Memorial Hospital.

Division of Allergy and Immunology, Department of Medicine, Northwestern University Feinberg School of Medicine, Suite 1000, 211 East Ontario Street, Chicago, IL 60611, USA

* Corresponding author.

E-mail address: l-grammer@northwestern.edu

Immunol Allergy Clin N Am 35 (2015) 349–362

http://dx.doi.org/10.1016/j.iac.2015.01.004
immunology.theclinics.com

be found for each case of anaphylaxis.[2] In addition, reports of IA were initially limited to the United States. However, in the 1990s, reports emerged from European countries, such as Spain, France, Ireland, Germany, and Brazil.[3] Subsequently, IA has become widely accepted as a disease process worthy of closer attention.

The pathophysiology of IA has not been fully elucidated, although elevated concentrations of urinary histamine and its metabolite, methylimidazole acetic acid, plasma histamine, and serum tryptase found in patients with this disorder is consistent with mast cell activation.[4] Manifestations of IA are identical to those episodes with a known cause. Despite early use of epinephrine autoinjector, some patients continue to experience life-threatening events, and there have been fatalities. There is a high prevalence of atopy in patients with IA with the rate found to be as high as 59% in one case series.[5] There is also a significantly higher prevalence in women compared with men.[6] However, after puberty and until menarche, the incidence has been reported to be similar in men and women.[6]

CLASSIFICATION

The classification of IA is based on frequency of episodes and clinical manifestations.[7] Frequent episodes are defined as having at least 2 episodes in the preceding 2 months or at least 6 episodes in the preceding year. Patients who do not meet either of these 2 criteria are categorized as having infrequent IA (**Table 1**). Generalized IA (IA-G) is characterized by urticaria and/or angioedema in addition to systemic symptoms, including cardiovascular, respiratory, and/or gastrointestinal symptoms. Some patients are categorized as IA-angioedema (IA-A), which is characterized by significant upper airway obstruction due to severe angioedema of the tongue, pharynx, or larynx without other signs of systemic anaphylaxis; patients may also have urticaria.

Table 1
Classification of idiopathic anaphylaxis

	Parameter	Comments
Classification	IA-G	Urticaria or angioedema with bronchospasm, hypotension, syncope
	IA-A	Angioedema with upper airway compromise (laryngeal, pharyngeal, tongue); may also have urticaria
Frequency	Frequent (F)	Definition: At least 2 episodes in the preceding 2 mo or at least 6 episodes in the preceding year
	Infrequent (I)	Definition: Fewer than 6 episodes a year
Severity	CSD-IA	Patient cannot be tapered off prednisone
	MCSD-IA	Patient requires at least 20 mg every day or 60 mg every other day prednisone to control IA
Variations of IA	IA-Q	Patient has possible IA but documentation of objective findings are unsuccessful and diagnosis is uncertain
	IA-V	Applied when symptoms of IA vary from classic IA
	Somatoform IA (IA-S)	Symptoms mimic IA but patients have no organic disease, documented objective findings, and are nonresponsive to the treatment regimen for IA

Adapted from Patterson R. Idiopathic anaphylaxis. East Providence (RI): OceanSide Publications, Inc; 1997. p. 20.

Some cases of IA are unclear and cannot be classified as either IA-G or IA-A. These cases are classified as IA-questionable (IA-Q), IA-variant (IA-V), or undifferentiated somatoform IA (US-IA). IA-Q describes patients who possibly have IA but do not have any documented objective finding and do not show a response to appropriate doses of prednisone. Thus, the diagnosis of IA remains unclear. IA-V describes patients whose symptoms and clinical findings differ from classic IA. US-IA is applied to patients who describe symptoms consistent with IA but have no organic disease or documented objective findings, are nonresponsive to the treatment regimen for IA, and meet DSM criteria for an undifferentiated somatoform disorder.[8] The patients with nonorganic disease present significant diagnostic and management issues and often cause considerable health care expenditure.[8]

In a study assessing the differences between IA-G and IA-A, a logistic regression model was constructed. Mast cell releasability was analyzed in the 2 groups using the log 10-wheal area produced by 4 consecutive concentrations of codeine. Using the logistic regression equation, IA-G and IA-A patients showed a higher cutaneous reaction to codeine than atopic patients. However, IA-G patients had a significantly lower reaction to codeine than those patients with chronic idiopathic urticaria.[9] No differences were observed in patients with IA-A compared with urticaria patients and there was no difference in cutaneous response to codeine between IA-A and IA-G patients.

EPIDEMIOLOGY

The precise prevalence of IA is unknown. Patterson and colleagues[10] performed a survey to estimate the prevalence of IA in the United States in 1995. In this survey, a questionnaire was mailed to all previous graduates of the Northwestern University Allergy and Immunology Fellowship program from the last 31 years. Of the 75 allergists surveyed, a total of 633 cases of IA were documented. By extrapolation of the cases of IA reported by the allergists surveyed to the approximately 4000 allergists in the United States at that time, it was estimated that the number of cases in the United States was between 20,592 and 47,024. In a recent study performed by Wood and colleagues,[11] 2 nationwide, cross-sectional random digit dial surveys were conducted in 2011. One of the surveys was a public survey of unselected adults and the other was a patient survey. Of the 1000 adult respondents, the prevalence of anaphylaxis in the general population was estimated at 1.6% or greater. Of these respondents, about 39% reported a possible idiopathic reaction. Webb and Lieberman[5] conducted a retrospective medical record review and follow-up questionnaires of anaphylaxis. The review spanned 25 years (1978–2003). Of the 601 cases, the highest percentage of patients (59%), was diagnosed with anaphylaxis because of unidentifiable causes. In a 3-year survey from the Mayo Clinic, 34 of 142 (24%) cases of anaphylaxis were reported to be idiopathic.[12]

The initial reports of IA were primarily in adults. Subsequently, this was recognized in pediatric populations. In children, the diagnosis of IA is delayed as compared with adults. There is often a history of multiple emergency room visits or hospitalizations before a diagnosis. Ditto and colleagues[13] published a case series of 22 pediatric patients with IA. They noted an increasing incidence of pediatric IA that they thought could be due to greater awareness that this condition does occur in the pediatric population.

The symptoms of anaphylaxis are similar to the adult population. In addition, the classification and treatment algorithm previously applied in the adult population are used in the pediatric population.[13,14] In a retrospective review of medical records of children presenting to a pediatric allergy clinic, 8 children diagnosed with IA were identified. The patients' ages ranged from 11 months to 19 years at disease onset. All these patients had cutaneous findings of urticaria, angioedema, or generalized flushing.

Many of the children had experienced life-threatening events, despite using epinephrine autoinjectors at onset of symptoms. In this study, there was a generally good response to appropriate therapy.[14]

Currently, there are ongoing efforts to improve the prevalence estimates of all forms of anaphylaxis. In a 2014 consensus document from the World Allergy Organization, the international research agenda for anaphylaxis included obtaining the global incidence and prevalence of anaphylaxis in general populations in different countries to obtain reliable population estimates.[15] The plan is to include data on anaphylaxis from all triggers and from specific triggers, including foods, stinging insects, other venoms and drugs with the goal being to collect data on anaphylaxis in different populations, such as infants, children, teenagers, pregnant women, the elderly, and patients with comorbidities such as asthma and cardiovascular disease. It is clear that regardless of the overall incidence of IA, it can have a significant, negative effect on quality of life as patients may have persistent anxiety about recurrent episodes and have neither a potential trigger to avoid nor a method to predict an episode.

POSSIBLE PATHOGENIC MECHANISMS

Numerous theories have been proposed to explain this condition. One theory involves an increase in the number of mast cells in patients with IA. Studies evaluating the number of mast cells in IA patients have found only a modest increase or no difference compared with healthy individuals.[16,17] In contrast with normal controls or IA patients, those with mastocytosis have a 10-fold increase in the density of cutaneous mast cells.

Another theory involves the release of mast cells or basophils. In a Spanish study, IA patients had more cutaneous reactivity to codeine than did atopic patients.[9] However, in a study conducted by Keffer and colleagues,[18] there was no difference in cutaneous response to intradermal morphine between IA patients and normal subjects. In addition, an in vitro study showed no difference in histamine release from peripheral blood basophils on stimulation with anti-immunoglobulin E (IgE) or with a calcium ionophore, A23187.[19]

In a case report published in 2007, a 30-year-old woman with multiple drug allergy syndrome who reported several episodes of anaphylaxis with angioedema and urticaria without any identifiable triggers for several episodes was found to have a positive in vivo autologous serum test and in vitro basophil histamine release assay.[20] This finding indicated the presence of circulating histamine-releasing factors. Thus, the authors proposed an autoreactive mechanism as the possible cause for IA.

Lymphocyte activation has been demonstrated in IA patients compared with normal patients. Grammer and colleagues[21] used flow cytometric analysis of lymphocyte markers to evaluate potential immunologic differences between normal control patients and IA patients in remission and during acute episodes. Total lymphocyte numbers were decreased in IA patients taking prednisone, consistent with known steroid effects on lymphocytes. Patients during acute episodes of IA were found to have statistically significant increases in T-cell activation markers compared with those in remission who had higher numbers of activated T cells compared with controls. No specific T-cell subset was identified as the primary subset involved in activation. Surprisingly, there was increased B-cell activation in IA patients, both during acute episodes and in remission, compared with control patients. The findings in this study would suggest that IA is an immunologic activation phenomenon consistent with the established clinical pattern of steroid responsive disease.

Other theories to explain IA include increased levels of anti-IgE autoantibodies, dysregulation of chemokines, such as uncontrolled production of histamine-release factors, or loss of histamine release inhibitory factors. It has been proposed that autoantibodies against IgE could cross-link IgE on mast cells and lead to the activation of mast cells and mediator release. In a pilot project, however, there was failure to detect anti-IgE antibodies in any of the 10 samples tested.[22]

In summary, many pathogenic mechanisms proposed to explain IA have not been supported by clinical and experimental studies.

CLINICAL MANIFESTATIONS

The signs and symptoms of patients diagnosed with IA are indistinguishable from the manifestations of other forms of anaphylaxis. The signs include angioedema, urticaria, wheezing, flushing, tachypnea, tachycardia, vomiting, diarrhea, syncope, hypotension, stridor, dysphagia, or hoarseness. The symptoms may include pruritus, dyspnea, lightheaded sensation, nausea, and abdominal pain/cramping, which can be severe, with urgent diarrhea. Urticaria is usually diffuse and severely pruritic and comprise erythematous well-circumscribed wheals with centers that blanch. Angioedema that frequently accompanies the urticaria usually presents in the form of swelling of the face, eyes, lips, genitals, or extremities. Angioedema may also affect the tongue, oropharynx, and larynx leading to severe life-threatening symptoms. The cardiac manifestations of anaphylaxis can be severe and are variable. Usually, tachycardia occurs as a compensatory mechanism for the decrease in effective vascular volume. Cardiovascular collapse may occur without any associated cutaneous or respiratory manifestations. Importantly, symptom onset may be sudden and progress at a rapid pace. Although some IA patients report that the time from onset of initial symptoms to life-threatening symptoms such as laryngeal edema, bronchospasm, and hypotension may be less than 10 minutes, others report several hours between symptom onset and anaphylaxis. In general, for a given patient, the timing and prodromal symptoms are similar with each episode. The first episode of IA usually is the worst, because the patient subsequently learns to recognize the prodromal symptoms and initiate emergency treatment in a timely fashion. Patients with rapid progression to life-threatening symptoms are at increased risk of more severe reactions in contrast with patients with slow progression of symptoms.

In a series of 335 patients diagnosed with IA, including both pediatric and adult patients, all had experienced angioedema and urticaria.[23] In addition, 210 (63%) experienced upper airway obstruction, 132 (39%) experienced bronchospasm, 78 (23%) experienced hypotension or syncope, and 75 (22%) experienced gastrointestinal symptoms. Angioedema of the gut can produce severe abdominal cramping, which is the prodrome in some patients. These patients have urgent bowel movements, most often diarrhea, with urticaria appearing while in the bathroom, followed by lightheadedness, and oftentimes, hypotension. In the authors' experience, some of these patients have been found unconscious on the bathroom floor by family or spouses.

DIFFERENTIAL DIAGNOSIS

The diagnosis of IA should be made only after exclusion of other potential causes of anaphylaxis and other diseases with similar manifestations to anaphylaxis (**Box 1**). Some common causes of anaphylaxis include foods and exercise-induced anaphylaxis (EIA). EIA usually occurs after vigorous exercise and is a result of mast cell activation. Symptoms may include urticaria, angioedema, nausea, vomiting,

Box 1
Differential diagnosis of idiopathic anaphylaxis

   i. Known causes of immediate generalized reactions

      A. IgE-mediated

         1. Foods

         2. Medications (2 examples listed)

            a. Penicillins

            b. Platins

         3. Food supplements (2 examples listed)

            a. Psyllium

            b. Bee pollen

      B. Exercise-induced anaphylaxis

      C. Food plus EIA

      D. Medication-induced reactions

         1. Aspirin

         2. NSAIDs

         3. Angiotensin-converting enzyme inhibitors

         4. Opiates

      E. Radiographic contrast media reactions

   ii. Hereditary angioedema (HAE)

      A. Classical form (also called type I)

         1. Absent C1 inhibitor

         2. Dysfunctional C1 inhibitor

      B. Acquired form (also called type II)

         1. B-cell lymphoproliferative disorder

         2. Autoantibodies to C1 inhibitor

      C. HAE with normal C1-INH (also called type III HAE)

  iii. Systemic mastocytosis

  iv. Asthma masquerading as anaphylaxis

   v. Munchausen stridor

  vi. Munchausen anaphylaxis

 vii. Undifferentiated somatoform IA

      A. Prevarication-anaphylaxis

      B. Simulated anaphylaxis

viii. Miscellaneous diagnoses

      A. Panic attacks

      B. Globus hystericus

      C. Vocal cord dysfunction

      D. Histamine-rich food induced flushing

      E. Carcinoid syndrome

      F. Pheochromocytoma

Adapted from Patterson R. Idiopathic anaphylaxis. East Providence (RI): OceanSide Publications, Inc; 1997. p. 20.

bronchospasm, laryngeal edema, respiratory distress, shock, and loss of consciousness. Some patients may have both IA and EIA. EIA may be unrelated to food, may occur only with a specific food, or may occur with any food ingestion. Medications are another common cause of anaphylactic reactions. Nonsteroidal anti-inflammatory drugs (NSAIDs), such as aspirin, may cause anaphylactic reactions through a non-IgE-medicated mechanism; there are also reports of IgE-mediated NSAID anaphylaxis. Although drugs such as β-lactams can cause IgE-mediated responses that occur within minutes to hours of ingestion, more severe reactions typically occur within 1 hour of ingestion or within minutes of parenteral administration.[24] Thus, a thorough medication history should be obtained from patients with anaphylaxis. Hereditary angioedema may also mimic anaphylaxis. It is characterized by recurrent episodes of angioedema usually involving the lips, tongue, or upper airway. The gastrointestinal tract may also be involved and may produce symptoms of cramping, abdominal pain, nausea, and diarrhea. Laboratory findings, including decreased levels of C4, CH50, and C1 esterase inhibitor level or function, may help differentiate this disorder from IA.

Some patients with pheochromocytoma and carcinoid syndrome may present with symptoms similar to symptoms of anaphylaxis. These patients often present with flushing as a result of release of vasoactive substances, such as epinephrine, norepinephrine, and vanillylmandelic acid in pheochromocytoma, and 5-hydroxyindoleacetic acid in carcinoid syndrome. Detection of these mediators via laboratory tests helps differentiate these disorders from IA. Severe asthma attacks may also be mistaken for IA. These patients may present with severe bronchoconstriction leading to dyspnea and wheezing, which can occur in IA patients. Symptoms limited to the lungs and prior history of hospitalizations for asthma would make a diagnosis of IA less likely.

Patients with Munchausen stridor complain of dyspnea and imitate stridulous sounds over the neck region. This stridorous respiration has no organic cause. These patients usually overuse epinephrine autoinjectors and emergency phone numbers and visit the emergency room frequently.[25] Patients with Munchausen stridor usually fail to respond to antihistamines or steroids.

Rare disorders that may mimic IA include delayed anaphylaxis to red meat. In contrast with immediate food-induced anaphylaxis, symptoms of urticaria or anaphylaxis may occur more than 2 hours after exposure. The relevant IgE antibody is specific for the oligosaccharide galactose-α-1,3-galactose, a blood group substance of non-primate mammals.[26] There is evidence that the primary cause of this IgE antibody response is tick bites. Diagnosis can be made by the presence of specific IgE to beef, lamb, pork, and milk and lack of IgE to turkey, chicken, or fish. Skin prick tests are usually negative, yet intradermals are usually positive.[26] Another infrequent cause of anaphylaxis is hydatid cyst rupture. A case of relapsing generalized anaphylactic reactions associated with life-threatening laryngospasm in a previously healthy man was published in a report from Germany. Workup revealed cystic liver echinococcosis with spontaneous rupture of the hydatid cyst.[27]

Other disorders included in the differential diagnosis of IA are systemic mastocytosis (SM), monoclonal mast cell activation syndrome, and mast cell activation syndrome. A certain subset of these patients has been shown to have evidence for clonal disorders of mast cells. In a study published by Akin and colleagues,[28] c-kit mutational analysis was positive in 3 of 12 patients with IA who did not exhibit either urticarial pigmentosa or characteristic bone marrow biopsy finding of multifocal mast cell aggregates observed in SM. Mast cell activation disorders are discussed in more detail elsewhere in this issue by Akin.

DIAGNOSTIC TESTS

The diagnosis of IA is one of exclusion. Thus, before arriving at this diagnosis, an extensive evaluation, including a thorough history, physical examination, and laboratory data, must be pursued. All hospitalization and emergency room records should be carefully examined for objective evidence of signs and symptoms, including hypotension, bronchospasm, and oropharyngeal angioedema. Particular attention must also be given to the treatment administered, response to treatment, and events surrounding the episode. Information on the severity and frequency of symptoms must also be obtained. The history should focus on the exclusion of potential allergens. Work and home environment history should include possible exposure to latex. The possibility of an association with insect stings, food or drug ingestion, and exercise (especially postprandial exercise) should be evaluated. Pigmented lesions that would suggest systemic mastocytosis must be excluded. If such lesions are present, then skin and bone marrow biopsies should be performed to confirm the diagnosis of mastocytosis. In rare cases, both upper and lower endoscopies may be performed to rule out a mastocytoma.

Laboratory data may include a complete blood cell count, chemistry panel, and liver function tests. Diagnostic tests to consider for a patient with unexplained anaphylaxis are listed in **Table 2**. Antinuclear antibody, erythrocyte sedimentation rate, and rheumatoid factor should be checked if a collagen vascular disorder is a possibility. Urinary histamine levels and serum tryptase levels may be useful because they may be elevated in generalized anaphylactic reactions. Spot urinary histamine levels or 24-hour urinary histamine levels remain elevated during attacks of IA.[29] Because of the short half-life and rapid release of plasma histamine, it is not ordinarily useful for diagnosis. Serum tryptase is generally more useful because the levels peak 60 to 90 minutes after onset of anaphylaxis; generally, the tryptase returns to normal within 6 hours, but there is a report of tryptase remaining elevated for 24 hours.[30] A systematic retrospective survey from 2006 to 2010 evaluating 171 patients with systemic reactions showed that a significant portion of patients with elevated acute serum tryptase levels had mild reactions that did not meet the World Allergy Organization criteria for anaphylaxis. Of note, 50% of the cases were diagnosed with IA. The correlation between acute serum tryptase level and severity of anaphylaxis was weak. This finding may reduce the specificity of the serum tryptase test.[31] Patients that have elevated tryptase both during acute attacks and at baseline should be evaluated for mastocytosis or other clonal mast cell disorders.

In a study of 102 patients with an initial diagnosis of IA evaluated with a battery of 79 selected food antigen skin prick tests, 32 (31%) had a positive test to one or more food antigens. In 5 of the patients, subsequently eating a food that was skin test positive provoked an anaphylactic reaction. Two patients completely eliminated the foods and ceased to experience reactions.[32] Thus, this may be a useful method for identifying an offending antigen in some cases. In another study, 110 patients with IA were tested with the Immuno Solid phase Allergen Chip (ISAC) allergen array containing 103 allergens. A wide range of major allergens was identified with ω-5-gliadin and shrimp, accounting for 45% of the previously unrecognized sensitizations. Twenty percent of the arrays were classified with a high likelihood of identifying the cause of anaphylaxis. The authors noted that the ISAC array contributed to the diagnosis in 20% of patients with IA.[33] Patients with IA may also have anaphylaxis because of known causes, including food, medications, or exercise.[19,23] It should also be noted that there are false positive food tests using either in vivo or in vitro tests for food-specific IgE, so testing should correlate with a history that is consistent with food allergy.

Table 2
Diagnostic tests to consider for a patient with unexplained anaphylaxis

Procedure	Comment
Urine histamine	To help confirm mast cell activation to secure the diagnosis
Serum tryptase	Supportive if elevated
Immediate skin testing for foods	May help to confirm or exclude food allergies as etiologic
Immediate skin testing for spices	To confirm or exclude an implicated spice
Immediate skin testing for penicillin	To confirm that penicillin was responsible for the anaphylaxis
Immediate skin testing for latex	May masquerade as idiopathic or food-induced anaphylaxis
Test dosing with NSAIDs	To demonstrate or exclude these as possible agents
Test dosing with a medication or food additive	To demonstrate or exclude these as causes for anaphylaxis
Complement determinations	To confirm or exclude C1 esterase inhibitor: deficiency/dysfunction C4, CH50
Bone marrow biopsy, skin biopsy, bone scan, liver scan	To exclude or confirm systemic mastocytosis or urticaria pigmentosa
Diagnostic therapeutic trial with prednisone for 2–3 mo	IA is prednisone responsive

Note: In vitro testing by RAST (radioallergosorbent test) or ELISA is less sensitive and can be less specific. Positive skin tests demonstrate IgE antibodies that may be related to episodes of anaphylaxis. However, they may occur in patients with IA and not make a diagnosis of an external cause for anaphylaxis.

Adapted from Patterson R. Idiopathic anaphylaxis. East Providence (RI): OceanSide Publications, Inc; 1997. p. 20.

TREATMENT

The treatment of IA is individualized based on the severity and frequency of a patient's symptoms. A general IA management algorithm appears in **Fig. 1**. Patients should receive instruction on the management of an acute episode. At the first sign of anaphylaxis, patients should administer 0.3 mL (1:1000) of aqueous epinephrine intramuscularly or subcutaneously, 60 mg of prednisone orally, and an oral H1 antihistamine. Hydroxyzine HC1 25 mg, diphenhydramine 50 mg, and chlorpheniramine 4 mg are the most studied, but second-generation antihistamines have also been used. Depending on the response to the initial injection, epinephrine administration may need to be repeated; this may be particularly true if the patient is taking β-blockers. However, these patients may also have a prominent α-adrenergic, hypertensive response. The patient should then proceed to the nearest emergency room in the safest and fastest way, which often means calling 911 for emergency medical services. Qualified personnel should follow Advanced Cardiac Life Support protocol. The patency of the airway must be assessed. If airway obstruction is severe and compromises ventilation, then intubation or tracheostomy may be necessary. Patients with severe hypotension may require rapid administration of intravenous crystalloid fluids preferably through 2 large-gauge venous catheters. Vasopressors such as dopamine or norepinephrine may be used for additional hemodynamic support, and epinephrine may need to be repeated or added as an infusion.

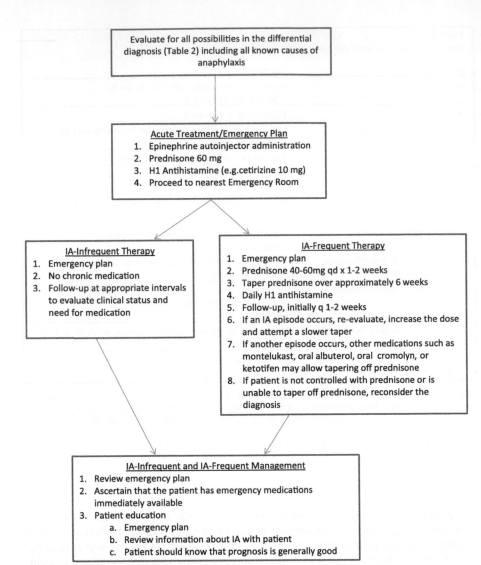

Fig. 1. IA management algorithm for the patient presenting with compatible history and objective signs of anaphylaxis.

Patients who experience frequent episodes are placed on prednisone to induce remission, at a dose 40 to 60 mg once daily for 1 week until symptoms are controlled, as well as an antihistamine (eg, hydroxyzine 25–50 mg 3 times daily or cetirizine 10 mg twice daily). However, higher doses of prednisone may be necessary in some patients. Daily dosing of prednisone for 1 to 2 weeks is usually required to achieve symptom control. If a longer daily prednisone course is required, the diagnosis of IA should be questioned. Once symptoms are stable, the dosing of prednisone may be converted to alternate day dosing. Prednisone should be tapered carefully (by 5 mg every other day every 1–2 weeks). Once prednisone is successfully tapered, the antihistamine may be gradually discontinued.[34]

Certain patients may be unable to discontinue prednisone because of recurrent symptoms. These patients have corticosteroid-dependent-IA (CSD-IA). If the prednisone dose required to control the IA is at least 20 mg every day or 60 mg every other day, the disease is termed malignant corticosteroid-dependent IA (MCSD-IA). In patients unable to taper off prednisone, drugs such as montelukast or an oral sympathomimetic such as albuterol could be used. Such patients may be given a trial of a mast cell stabilizer such as oral cromolyn (especially if gastrointestinal symptoms are prominent) or ketotifen. If the prednisone requirement does not change once the mast cell stabilizer is added, the drug should be discontinued because there has been no benefit. Of note, oral ketotifen is not commercially available in the United States. This treatment may allow tapering and eventual discontinuation of steroids, thus achieving a remission.[35] In a series of 5 patients with either severe IA or CSD-IA, all 5 patients had a reduction or resolution of their episodes of IA while on ketotifen. If a patient does not respond to the outlined IA treatment, the diagnosis must be seriously re-evaluated and the diagnoses in **Box 1** should be reconsidered.

Omalizumab has also been found to induce remission in an IA patient who was recalcitrant to other therapies.[36] There are other case reports in the literature documenting similar results with omalizumab.[37]

Patients with IA-infrequent generally do not require maintenance therapy unless the most recent episode was considered very severe or if the patient has significant comorbidities putting them at risk of hypotension, arrhythmias, and so on. Patient education and an emergency action plan are very important elements of their treatment.

Patients who have experienced anaphylactic episodes should be offered the option of wearing jewelry or carrying identification cards stating their diagnosis of IA. Patients who are taking β-blockers and ACE inhibitors are at increased risk of treatment-resistant anaphylaxis. If possible, those drugs should be avoided in IA patients. Education remains the major goal in the prevention and management of serious episodes of IA. Patients should be well versed regarding the emergency treatment plan for acute episodes, including injectable epinephrine syringes, prednisone, antihistamine, as well as in seeking further care at the nearest emergency department.

PROGNOSIS

The prognosis of IA is generally favorable. In a retrospective study of 37 patients with IA ranging from 26 to 71 years, frequent episodes of IA defined as greater than 5 episodes per year occurred in 31% at presentation.[12] At follow-up, 21 patients (60%) had resolution of IA and the frequency of anaphylaxis decreased in 9 patients, increased in 2 patients, and remained the same in 3 patients. Only 3 patients were still experiencing frequent episodes and only 2 required chronic glucocorticoids. Patients with frequent IA treated with only antihistamines achieved remission or improvement at the same rate as those treated with chronic steroids.[12] In studies from Northwestern University, the overwhelming majority of patients achieve remission.[13,19,23] If a remission cannot be achieved, other diagnoses should be reconsidered. Recurrence of anaphylaxis in idiopathic anaphylactic patients does occur. In a study by Alonso and colleagues[38] assessing the risk of recurrence of different subtypes of anaphylaxis, recurrence of anaphylaxis was higher for idiopathic, foods, and exercise compared with other subtypes of anaphylaxis, such as medications and hymenoptera stings. The total incidence of recurrence was 3.2 episodes per 100 person-years, whereas the incidence of recurrence for IA subtype was 4.9 episodes per 100 person-years. Thus, if a cause has been identified, particular care should be given to prevention in this population with recurrent anaphylaxis.

Despite appropriate treatment, fatalities from IA can occur. Krasnick and colleagues[39] reported one fatality. However, the authors note that compliance with prednisone was not certain because the patient had reported dislike of prednisone to his friends. In addition, the patient had asthma, which has been associated with an increased risk of fatal anaphylactic reactions.

SUMMARY

- IA is a diagnosis of exclusion after other causes, such as foods, medications, exercise, insect stings, C1 esterase inhibitor deficiency, and mastocytosis, have been excluded. The signs and symptoms of patients diagnosed with IA are indistinguishable from the manifestations of other forms of anaphylaxis.
- A significant proportion (24%–59%) of anaphylaxis cases are classified as idiopathic in several reported patient series. There is a higher prevalence of IA in women compared with men. There is also a high prevalence of atopy in patients with IA. IA is less common in children but does occur.
- The classification of IA is based on frequency of episodes and clinical manifestations. Frequent episodes are defined as at least 2 episodes in the preceding 2 months or at least 6 episodes in the preceding year. Patients who do not meet either of these 2 criteria are categorized as infrequent.
- The treatment of IA is individualized based on the severity and frequency of a patient's symptoms. The acute treatment of IA is the same as treatment of anaphylaxis from other causes, except that prolonged tapering of prednisone is usually required to induce remission. All patients should possess an epinephrine autoinjector and an anaphylaxis emergency plan.
- The prognosis of IA is generally favorable with appropriate treatment and patient education.

REFERENCES

1. Bacal E, Patterson R, Zeiss CR. Evaluation of severe (anaphylactic) reactions. Clin Allergy 1978;8:295–304.
2. Patterson R. Idiopathic anaphylaxis. Providence (RI): Oceanside Publications, Inc; 1997.
3. Lieberman PL. Idiopathic anaphylaxis. Allergy Asthma Proc 2013;35:17–23.
4. Tanus T, Mines D, Atkins PC, et al. Serum tryptase in idiopathic anaphylaxis: a case report and review of the literature. Ann Emerg Med 1994;24:104–7.
5. Webb L, Lieberman P. Anaphylaxis: a review of 601 cases. Ann Allergy Asthma Immunol 2006;97:39–43.
6. Moneret-Vautrin DA, Gay G. The so-called "idiopathic anaphylaxis": allergic and pseudo-allergic reactions. Allerg Immunol (Paris) 1991;23:89–93 [in French].
7. Greenberger PA. Idiopathic anaphylaxis. Immunol Allergy Clin North Am 2007; 27:273.
8. Choy C, Patterson R, Patterson DR, et al. Undifferentiated somatoform idiopathic anaphylaxis: nonorganic symptoms mimicking idiopathic anaphylaxis. J Allergy Clin Immunol 1995;96:893–900.
9. Tejedor A, Dominguez S, Sanchez-Hernandez J, et al. Clinical and functional differences among patients with idiopathic anaphylaxis. J Investig Allergol Clin Immunol 2004;14(3):177–86.
10. Patterson R, Hogan M, Yarnold P, et al. Idiopathic anaphylaxis. Arch Intern Med 1995;155:869–71.

11. Wood R, Camargo C, Lieberman P, et al. Anaphylaxis in America: the prevalence and characteristics of anaphylaxis in the United States. J Allergy Clin Immunol 2014;133:461–7.
12. Khan DA, Yocum MW. Clinical course of idiopathic anaphylaxis. Ann Allergy 1994;73:370–4.
13. Ditto AM, Krasnick J, Greenberger P, et al. Pediatric idiopathic anaphylaxis: experience with 22 patients. J Allergy Clin Immunol 1997;100:320–6.
14. Hogan MB, Kelly MA, Wilson NW. Idiopathic anaphylaxis in children. Ann Allergy Asthma Immunol 1998;81:140–2.
15. Simons FE, Ardusso L, Bilo M, et al. International consensus on (ICON) anaphylaxis. World Allergy Organ J 2014;7:9.
16. Garriga MM, Firedman MM, Metcalfe DD. A survey of the number and distribution of mast cells in the skin of patients with mast cell disorders. J Allergy Clin Immunol 1988;82(3):425–32.
17. Irani AA, Garriga MM, Metcalfe DD, et al. Mast cells in cutaneous mastocytosis: accumulation of the MCTC type. Clin Exp Allergy 1990;20:53–8.
18. Keffer J, Bressler RB, Wright R, et al. Analysis of the wheal and flare reactions that follow the intradermal injection of histamine and morphine in adults with recurrent unexplained anaphylaxis and systemic mastocytosis. J Allergy Clin Immunol 1989;83:595.
19. Sonin L, Grammer LC, Greenberger PA, et al. Idiopathic anaphylaxis: a clinical summary. Ann Intern Med 1983;99:634.
20. Tedeschi A, Lorini M, Suli C, et al. Detection of serum histamine-releasing factors in a patient with idiopathic anaphylaxis and multiple drug allergy syndrome. J Investig Allergol Clin Immunol 2007;17(2):122–5.
21. Grammer LC, Shaughnessy MA, Harris KE, et al. Lymphocyte subsets and activation markers in patients with acute episodes of idiopathic anaphylaxis. Ann Allergy Asthma Immunol 2000;85:368–71.
22. Gruber BL, Baeza ML, Marchese MJ, et al. Prevalence and functional role of anti-IgE autoantibodies in urticarial syndromes. J Invest Dermatol 1988;90:213.
23. Ditto AM, Harris KE, Krasnick J, et al. Idiopathic anaphylaxis: a series of 335 cases. Ann Allergy Asthma Immunol 1996;77:285–91.
24. Pumphrey RS. Lessons for management of anaphylaxis from a study of fatal reactions. Clin Exp Allergy 2000;30:114–50.
25. Bahna SL, Oldham JL. Munchausen stridor—a strong false alarm of anaphylaxis. Allergy Asthma Immunol Res 2014;6:577–9.
26. Tripathi A, Commins SP, Heymann PW, et al. Delayed anaphylaxis to red meat masquerading as idiopathic anaphylaxis. J Allergy Clin Immunol Pract 2014; 2(3):259–65.
27. Stey C, Jost R, Ammann R. Recurrent life-threatening anaphylaxis as initial manifestation of cystic echinococcosis (granulosus) of the liver. Schweiz Med Wochenschr 1993;123(29):1445–7.
28. Akin C, Scott L, Kocabas C. Demonstration of an aberrant mast cell population with clonal markers in a subset of patients with idiopathic anaphylaxis. Blood 2007;110(7):233.
29. Kaliner M, Dyer J, Merlins S, et al. Increased urinary histamine in contrast media reactions. Invest Radiol 1984;19:116.
30. Shanmugam G, Schwartz LB, Khan DA. Prolonged elevation of serum tryptase in idiopathic anaphylaxis. J Allergy Clin Immunol 2006;117:950–1.
31. Sristava S, Huissoon AP, Barrett V, et al. Systemic reactions and anaphylaxis with an acute serum tryptase ≥14 µg/L: retrospective characterisation of aetiology,

severity and adherence to National Institute of Health and Care Excellence (NICE) guidelines for serial tryptase measurements and specialist referral. J Clin Pathol 2014;67:614–9.

32. Stricker WE, Anorve Lopez E, Reed CE. Food skin testing in patients with idiopathic anaphylaxis. J Allergy Clin Immunol 1986;77(3):516–9.

33. Heaps A, Carter S, Selwood C, et al. The utility of the ISAC allergen array in the investigation of idiopathic anaphylaxis. Clin Exp Immunol 2014;177(2):483–90.

34. Patterson R, Stoloff RF, Greenberger PA, et al. Algorithms for the diagnosis and management of idiopathic anaphylaxis. Ann Allergy 1993;71:40–4.

35. Patterson R, Fitzsimons EJ, Choy C, et al. Malignant and corticosteroid-dependent idiopathic anaphylaxis: successful responses to ketotifen. Ann Allergy Asthma Immunol 1997;79:138–44.

36. Jones JD, Marney SR, Fahrenholz JM. Idiopathic anaphylaxis successfully treated with omalizumab. Ann Allergy Asthma Immunol 2008;101:550–1.

37. Lee J. Successful prevention of recurrent anaphylactic events with anti-immunoglobulin E therapy. Asia Pac Allergy 2014;4:126–8.

38. Alonso T, Garcia M, Hernandez J. Recurrence of anaphylaxis in a Spanish series. J Investig Allergol Clin Immunol 2013;23(6):383–91.

39. Krasnick J, Patterson R, Meyers G. A fatality from idiopathic anaphylaxis. Ann Allergy Asthma Immunol 1996;76:376–9.

Recognition, Treatment, and Prevention of Anaphylaxis

Lindsey E. Moore, DO[a], Ann M. Kemp, RPh, MD[b],
Stephen F. Kemp, MD[a],*

KEYWORDS

- Anaphylaxis • Epinephrine • Management • Observation • Prevention

KEY POINTS

- Anaphylaxis remains a clinical diagnosis based on probability and pattern recognition.
- The evidence base for the treatment of anaphylaxis is weak and largely based on consensus expert recommendations and anecdotal reports.
- Intramuscular epinephrine is the treatment of choice for acute anaphylaxis.
- Education, avoidance, and prevention are critically important because some anaphylactic reactions are so severe that death occurs despite rapid recognition and treatment.

INTRODUCTION

Anaphylaxis, an acute and potentially lethal multisystem allergic reaction, occurs in a variety of clinical scenarios and is almost unavoidable. Immunologic reactions to medications, foods, and insect stings cause most episodes, but virtually any substance capable of inducing systemic degranulation of mast cells and basophils can produce anaphylaxis. International studies suggest the lifetime prevalence is 0.05% to 2% with a mortality of 1%.[1,2] An expedient diagnosis of anaphylaxis can be challenging. Prevention of future episodes involves collaborative efforts between patients and their family members, community, and health care professionals. This article focuses on current recommendations for the recognition, treatment, and prevention of anaphylaxis.

Conflicts of interest: Dr S.F. Kemp has served as an anaphylaxis advisor for Sanofi US Services (Bridgewater, NJ). The other authors have no potential conflicts of interest to declare.
[a] Division of Clinical Immunology and Allergy, Department of Medicine, The University of Mississippi Medical Center, Jackson, MS 39216, USA; [b] Department of Family Medicine, The University of Mississippi Medical Center, Jackson, MS 39216, USA
* Corresponding author. Division of Clinical Immunology and Allergy, Department of Medicine, The University of Mississippi Medical Center, 878 Lakeland Drive, Building LB, Jackson, MS 39216.
E-mail address: skemp@umc.edu

CLINICAL RECOGNITION OF ANAPHYLAXIS

Anaphylaxis remains a clinical diagnosis based on pattern recognition and probability. No evaluation can prove causation of anaphylaxis conclusively without directly challenging the patient with the suspected agent, which is a course of action that is generally contraindicated by ethical and safety concerns. Cause and effect often are confirmed historically in patients who experience objective findings of anaphylaxis after inadvertent reexposure to the causal agent.

As highlighted in symposia jointly sponsored by the National Institute of Allergy and Infectious Diseases and the Food Allergy and Anaphylaxis Network, anaphylaxis is defined as a "serious allergic reaction that is rapid in onset and may cause death" and is considered likely if any 1 of 3 criteria is satisfied within minutes to hours: (1) acute onset of illness with involvement of skin, mucosal surface, or both, and at least 1 of the following: respiratory compromise, hypotension, or end-organ dysfunction; (2) 2 or more of the following occur rapidly after exposure to a likely allergen: involvement of skin or mucosal surface, respiratory compromise, hypotension, or persistent gastrointestinal symptoms; (3) hypotension develops after exposure to a known allergen for that patient: age-specific low blood pressure or decreased systolic blood pressure more than 30% compared with baseline.[3] A retrospective cohort study of 214 emergency department patients ascertained that these criteria had a positive predictive value of 69% and a negative predictive value of 98%.[4] However, anaphylaxis occurs as part of a clinical continuum that can begin with minor symptoms such as itchy skin, eyes, or nose and rapidly progress to life-threatening respiratory or cardiovascular manifestations. In clinical practice, the ultimate severity of an anaphylactic reaction is difficult to predict at its onset.

Anaphylaxis is associated with 1 or more of the following signs and symptoms: diffuse erythema and pruritus, urticaria, angioedema, bronchospasm, laryngeal edema, hyperperistalsis (eg, abdominal cramps, emesis, diarrhea), uterine cramps, hypotension, or cardiac arrhythmias. Urticaria and angioedema are the most common manifestations, but cutaneous findings may be delayed or absent in rapidly progressive anaphylaxis or they may vary with certain populations (eg, in children or in perioperative anaphylaxis).[2,5] The next most common manifestations of anaphylaxis are respiratory symptoms, followed by dizziness, syncope, and gastrointestinal symptoms. The more rapid the occurrence of anaphylaxis after exposure to a stimulus, the more likely the reaction is to be severe and potentially life threatening.[1,2]

Anaphylactic reactions may be immediate and uniphasic or they may be delayed in onset, biphasic (recurrent), or protracted. The reported time of onset of the late phase of biphasic anaphylaxis varies from 1 to 72 hours after apparent resolution of the initial phase.[6,7] Protracted anaphylaxis may persist for up to 32 hours.[7] Neither biphasic nor protracted anaphylaxis can be predicted from the severity of the initial phase of an anaphylactic reaction because they have occurred after what were perceived initially to be mild episodes.

MANAGEMENT OF ANAPHYLAXIS

Systematic reviews have noted the lack of optimal, randomized controlled trials of epinephrine, antihistamines, and glucocorticoids in anaphylaxis.[8–11] Pending a stronger evidence base for the treatment of anaphylaxis, practice parameters and consensus emergency management guidelines afford the best clinical guidance.[12–15] However, physicians and other health care professionals may not follow them.[16–18]

Clinicians who perform procedures and administer medications should have the appropriate medications and equipment available to treat anaphylaxis.[2,12,15] A sequential approach to the management of anaphylaxis is outlined in **Box 1**. The prompt,

---

Box 1
Management of acute anaphylaxis

1. Immediate intervention:

   a. Assessment of airway, breathing, circulation, and adequacy of mentation

   b. Administer IM epinephrine every 5 to 15 minutes, as necessary, to control anaphylaxis signs and symptoms and prevent progression to more severe symptoms (eg, respiratory distress, hypotension, and unconsciousness)

   c. Place patient in recumbent position and elevate lower extremities, as tolerated

2. Subsequent measures depending on response to IM epinephrine:

   a. Consider call for assistance and transportation to an emergency department or an intensive care facility

   b. Establish and maintain airway

   c. Administer oxygen

   d. Establish venous access

   e. Use IV (IO) crystalloid (eg, 0.9% saline or Ringer's lactate) for fluid replacement

3. Specific measures to consider after epinephrine injections, where appropriate:

   a. Consider dilute epinephrine infusion

   b. Consider H_1 and H_2 antihistamines

   c. Consider nebulized beta2-agonist (eg, albuterol) for bronchospasm resistant to epinephrine

   d. Consider systemic glucocorticoids

   e. Consider vasopressor (eg, dopamine)

   f. Consider glucagon for patient taking β-blocker

4. Observation and subsequent outpatient follow-up:

   a. Observation periods after apparent resolution must be individualized

   b. After recovery from the acute episode, every patient should receive epinephrine autoinjectors and be instructed in proper technique

   c. Every patient after anaphylaxis requires a careful diagnostic evaluation in consultation with an allergist-immunologist

Abbreviations: IM, intramuscular; IO, intraosseous; IV, intravenous.
   Data from Lieberman P, Nicklas RA, Oppenheimer J, et al. Joint Task Force on Practice Parameters. The diagnosis and management of anaphylaxis practice parameter: 2010 update. J Allergy Clin Immunol 2010;126:480, e32.

---

judicious use of intramuscular epinephrine and the maintenance of airway, adequate oxygenation, and effective circulatory volume are paramount considerations. Patients should be monitored continuously to facilitate prompt detection of any new clinical findings or treatment complications. When a patient should be transferred to an emergency facility depends on the severity of the anaphylaxis, the response to treatment, the expertise of the individual clinician, the estimated time of arrival of assistance, and possibly other scenario-dependent factors.

Epinephrine

Epinephrine is the treatment of choice for anaphylaxis and should be administered as soon as the clinician makes the clinical diagnosis of anaphylaxis (**Table 1**; Kemp and

Table 1
Therapeutic agents for anaphylaxis

Intervention	Dose and Route of Administration	Comments
Epinephrine 1:1000 v/v (1 mg/mL)	0.2–0.5 mg IM thigh (adult); 0.01 mg/kg (up to 0.3 mg) IM thigh (child)	Give immediately; repeat every 5–15 min as needed. Monitor for toxicity
Epinephrine infusion	1 mg of 1:1000 v/v (1 mg/mL) dilution added to 250 mL D5W (or NS) (ie, 4 μg/mL concentration) infused at 1–4 μg/min (15–60 drops/min with microdrop), increasing to maximum 10 μg/min	Give if hypotensive shock and no response to IM epinephrine and IV (IO) fluids; titrate to blood pressure response. Continuous use requires critical care monitoring. Monitor for toxicity
Volume Expansion		
Normal saline Ringer's lactate	Adult, 1–2 L rapidly IV/IO (5–10 mL/kg in first 5 min); child,[a] 20 mL/kg in first hr	Rate is titrated to blood pressure and pulse rate. Insert the largest catheter possible into the largest, most secure peripheral vein available. Use an administration set that permits rapid infusions. Monitor for volume overload
Antihistamines		
Diphenhydramine	Adult, 25–50 mg IV (IO); child,[a] 1 mg/kg IV (IO) up to 50 mg infused over 10 min	Second-line agents: H1 and H2 agents might work better in combination than H1 agents alone in urticarial suppression. Standard oral doses might suffice in milder episodes
Ranitidine	Adult, 50 mg IV (IO) (adults); child,[a] 12.5–50 mg, infused over 10 min	—
Glucocorticoids		
Methylprednisolone	1–2 mg/kg/d IV (IO)	Second-line agents: exact dose not established; no role in acute anaphylaxis
Prednisone	0.5 mg/kg/d PO	—
Vasopressor		
Dopamine	400 mg in 500 mL D5W (or NS) infused at 2–5 μg/kg/min	Consider if hypotensive and no response to epinephrine and fluids; titrate to maintain blood pressure; continuous use requires critical care monitoring
Glucagon	Initial dose, 1–5 mg slow IV (IO), then 5–15 μg/min infusion	Consider if treatment complicated by β-adrenergic blockade; emesis precautions needed; titrate to blood pressure
Methylene blue	Single bolus, 1.5–2 mg/kg in 100 mL D5W infused over 20 min has been used	Optimal dose unknown; should avoid in patients with G6PD deficiency, pulmonary hypertension, acute lung injury

Abbreviations: D5W, 5% dextrose in water; G6PD, glucose-6-phosphodiesterase; IM, intramuscular; IO, intraosseous; IV, intravenous; NS, normal saline; PO, orally; v/v, volume/volume.

[a] Child dosage is age independent and determined by prepubertal state and weight less than 40 kg.

Adapted from Kemp SF. Office approach to anaphylaxis: sooner better than later. Am J Med 2007;120:666; and Kemp AM, Kemp SF. Pharmacotherapy in refractory anaphylaxis: when intramuscular epinephrine fails. Curr Opin Allergy Clin Immunol 2014;14:375.

colleagues[19] discuss some of the complexities involved in decision making).[3,12–15,20–22] Westfall and Westfall[23] provide a detailed review of the pharmacology of epinephrine. Note that there is no absolute contraindication for epinephrine administration in anaphylaxis.[12,19] All subsequent therapeutic interventions depend on the initial response to this medication.[12,19] Fatalities from anaphylaxis can result from delayed or inadequate doses of epinephrine and from severe respiratory or cardiovascular complications.[12,24] Delayed epinephrine administration might also contribute to the likelihood of biphasic anaphylaxis.[6,7,12] Even with optimal treatment, some patients still die from anaphylaxis.[2,12,15,24]

The α-adrenergic, vasoconstrictive effects of recommended dosages of intramuscular epinephrine reverse peripheral vasodilation and alleviate hypotension and reduce generalized cutaneous erythema, urticaria, and angioedema. Local injection of epinephrine might reduce further absorption of antigen from a sting or injection site, but this has not been studied systematically. The β-adrenergic properties of epinephrine cause bronchodilation, increase myocardial output and contractility, and suppress further mediator release from mast cells and basophils.[19,23]

Epinephrine administration enhances coronary blood flow. Two mechanisms are probably responsible: an increased duration of myocardial diastole compared with systole and a vasodilator effect caused by increased contractility. These actions usually offset the vasoconstrictor effects of epinephrine on the coronary arteries.[19,23]

Common pharmacologic effects of epinephrine that occur at recommended doses via any route of administration include agitation, anxiety, tremulousness, headache, dizziness, pallor, or palpitations.[19,23] Rarely, and usually after excessive doses, epinephrine administration might contribute to or cause myocardial ischemia or infarction, pulmonary edema, prolonged QTc interval, ventricular arrhythmias, accelerated or malignant states of hypertension, and intracranial hemorrhage. Nonetheless, some patients have survived massive doses of epinephrine without evident myocardial ischemia or residual complications.[19]

The evidence base supporting the prompt use of epinephrine in anaphylaxis is less robust than the evidence base for treatment used in other common medical conditions (eg, asthma) and likely will remain so for ethical, clinical, and logistic considerations.[8,11,15,25] A systematic review concluded that, despite suboptimal evidence, intramuscular injections of epinephrine remain the treatment of choice for anaphylaxis.[8]

THERAPEUTIC OPTIONS AFTER INTRAMUSCULAR EPINEPHRINE
Oxygen and Beta2-agonists

Practice parameters and international guidelines support the use of oxygen and beta2-agonists in anaphylaxis, but no high-quality studies have evaluated their implementation.[11–14,21,22,26] Thus, oxygen should be administered and pulse oximetry monitored during anaphylaxis for patients who require multiple doses of epinephrine, have protracted anaphylaxis, or have preexisting hypoxemia or myocardial dysfunction. The rate of oxygen flow depends on the clinical response and the device used. A nasal cannula at 4 to 6 L/min delivers 25% to 40% oxygen, whereas a simple face mask at 8 to 12 L/min delivers 50% to 60% oxygen.[12]

Patients with epinephrine-resistant bronchospasm usually respond to inhaled beta2-agonists (eg, albuterol) delivered with oxygen nebulization. Recommended dosages are extrapolated from asthma management guidelines.

Fluid Resuscitation for Persistent Hypotension

Increased vascular permeability during anaphylaxis can shift up to 35% of intravascular volume into the extravascular compartment within 10 minutes, potentially resulting in inadequate venous return to the heart.[27,28] Placement in the recumbent position with the legs elevated, as tolerated, thus is highly recommended in anaphylaxis, and it is essential in hypotensive patients because it provides autotransfusion of approximately 1 to 2 L of fluid into the central vascular compartment.[29]

No high-quality studies have evaluated the therapeutic use of intravenous fluids in anaphylaxis and there is insufficient conclusive evidence from various other clinical conditions to provide general guidance for the optimal administration of isotonic crystalloid fluid resuscitation.[11,30] A Canadian survey observed that the selection of 0.9% saline versus lactated Ringer's solution varies by specialty; internists tend to prefer the former, whereas surgeons and anesthesiologists tend to prefer the latter.[31] Aggressive use of 0.9% saline potentially risks hyperchloremic metabolic acidosis, whereas large volumes of lactated Ringer's potentially risk respiratory acidosis.[32]

Practice parameters and international guidelines promote the use of the crystalloid solution, 0.9% saline, for epinephrine-resistant hypotension in anaphylaxis (see **Table 1**).[12–15,20,26] Large volumes might be required (eg, 7 L).[2,12] If multiple liters of saline are necessary, 0.45% saline can be substituted to help prevent hyperchloremic metabolic acidosis. A critical care setting permits monitoring of electrolytes as part of the emergency care.

Any drug or fluid that is administered intravenously can also be given intraosseously in any age group.[33] Thus, clinicians who are proficient at obtaining intraosseous cannulation might consider it if intravenous access is delayed or unsuccessful because it provides safe and efficacious access to a noncollapsible venous plexus.

Intravenous Epinephrine

No scientifically rigorous studies presently permit recommendations concerning the use of intravenous epinephrine in anaphylaxis.[11] However, parameters and international guidelines support its use in refractory anaphylaxis (see **Table 1**).[12–15] Because of the risk for potentially lethal arrhythmias, epinephrine characteristically is administered intravenously only in patients with cardiac arrest or to unresponsive or hypotensive patients who fail to respond to fluid resuscitation and multiple epinephrine injections.[2,12] One group of investigators suggests that the early use of intravenous epinephrine is effective and well tolerated when the rate of administration is titrated to the clinical response, but no cohort study has systematically compared this modality with intramuscular injections of epinephrine.[2,34] Continuous hemodynamic monitoring is optimal, but its absence should not preclude the use of intravenous epinephrine if considered essential after several epinephrine injections. In this special circumstance, monitoring by available means (eg, every-minute measurements of pulse rate and blood pressure) should be considered.[12]

SECOND-LINE THERAPEUTIC AGENTS FOR ANAPHYLAXIS

Parameters and international guidelines support the consideration of antihistamines, glucocorticoids, vasopressors, and glucagon for the treatment of anaphylaxis after initial use of epinephrine and fluids (see **Table 1**).[12–15,20–22] However, the quality of evidence is presently insufficient to permit recommendations concerning their use.[9–11,35–37]

Antihistamines

Skidgel and colleagues[38] provide a detailed review of H_1 and H_2 antihistamine pharmacology. Antihistamines act much more slowly than epinephrine; they have minimal favorable influence on blood pressure and they should not be administered alone for anaphylaxis treatment.[12] Even at maximum dosages, they cannot abort anaphylaxis if other inflammatory mediators are involved. However, antihistamines can attenuate cutaneous manifestations (eg, urticaria or pruritus). Intravenous administration ensures that effective dosing will not be diminished by hemodynamic compromise, which impairs gastrointestinal or intramuscular absorption, but maximal therapeutic effect might not be observed for 1 hour.[39] Caution should be taken, because intravenously administered H_1 antihistamines can also cause hypotension.[40]

Few guidelines support consideration of H_2 antihistamines in anaphylaxis after the initial use of epinephrine and fluids.[12–14,21] Ranitidine is usually recommended when H_2 antihistamines are considered in anaphylaxis. Hypotension may result from rapid intravenous administration of cimetidine.[12]

Glucocorticoids

Schimmer and Funder[41] provide a detailed review of the pharmacology of glucocorticoids. Systemic glucocorticoids may not exert appreciable effects for several hours, but they might prevent biphasic or protracted reactions in some patients. However, the data concerning possible preventive benefits are conflicting and limited.[6,7,35] Patients with asthma or other conditions recently treated with glucocorticoids might be at an increased risk for severe or fatal anaphylaxis and might receive additional benefit if glucocorticoids are administered to them during anaphylaxis. Recommended dosages are extrapolated from acute asthma management.

Vasopressors

Vasopressors (eg, dopamine) are reserved for the rare occurrence when epinephrine and fluids both fail to alleviate hypotension in anaphylaxis.[2,12–15] A critical care specialist may be needed for these events. A systematic review concluded that the effect of vasopressors on patient-relevant outcomes in hypotensive shock remains controversial and thus evidence-based recommendations to support one investigated vasopressor rather than another are not possible.[36]

Glucagon

Usual doses of epinephrine administered during anaphylaxis may not have the desired clinical effect in patients taking β-blockers and may instead exert predominately α-adrenergic effects. In such circumstances, isotonic volume expansion and glucagon administration are both recommended.[12,15,37] By directly activating adenyl cyclase, glucagon bypasses the β-adrenergic receptor and thus may reverse refractory hypotension and bronchospasm associated with anaphylaxis, as shown in limited case reports.[37] Airway protection is especially important in severely drowsy patients because glucagon can cause emesis and increase the risk for aspiration.

Methylene Blue

Parameters and international guidelines briefly mention methylene blue, which might be an emerging consideration as a second-line therapeutic agent for anaphylaxis (see **Table 1**).[12,20] Seven case reports describe the use of methylene blue for the treatment of anaphylactic shock refractory to epinephrine, intravenous fluids, vasopressors, and intra-aortic balloon pump, and 1 report describes its successful use in a normotensive patient with refractory anaphylaxis.[42–44] The optimal dosage for use in anaphylaxis has not been determined. Methylene blue presumably exerts its therapeutic effects by blocking nitric oxide–mediated relaxation of vascular smooth muscle. However, the administration of methylene blue itself can precipitate anaphylaxis in some individuals.[45,46]

OBSERVATION AFTER ANAPHYLAXIS

The best evidence suggests that observation periods after complete resolution of uniphasic anaphylaxis should be individualized, particularly because there are no reliable predictors of biphasic anaphylaxis. An observation period based on the severity and response to treatment is appropriate. Initial phases of anaphylaxis characterized by hypotension, respiratory failure or hypoxemia, repeated doses of epinephrine, poorly controlled asthma, or prior history of biphasic anaphylaxis are reasonable indications for an observation period of at least 24 hours. At discharge, all patients should be provided epinephrine autoinjectors and receive proper instruction on how to self-administer them in case of a subsequent episode. Patients should also have ready access to emergency medical services for prompt transportation to the closest emergency department for treatment. Further prospective studies on biphasic anaphylaxis are needed.[6,7,12,14,47]

PREVENTION OF ANAPHYLAXIS

Education, avoidance, and prevention are critically important because some anaphylactic reactions are so severe that death occurs despite rapid recognition and treatment. **Box 2** outlines basic principles for the prevention of future anaphylaxis. An allergist-immunologist can provide comprehensive professional advice on these matters.

Box 2
Preventive measures in anaphylaxis

General measures

- Obtain thorough history to identify the causes of anaphylaxis and those individuals at risk for future attacks

- Provide instruction on proper reading of food and medication labels, where appropriate

- Avoid drugs immunologically or biochemically cross reactive with any agents to which the patient is sensitive

- Manage comorbid conditions

- Administer drugs orally rather than parenterally, when possible

- Implement a waiting period of 20 to 30 minutes after injections of drugs or other biologic agents

- Consider a waiting period of 2 hours if a patient receives a particular oral medication for the first time in the office

- Consult allergist-immunologist for assistance

Specific measures for high-risk patients

- Individuals at high risk for anaphylaxis should carry epinephrine autoinjectors at all times and receive instruction in proper use with placebo trainer (includes patients receiving monoclonal antibody therapy)

- MedicAlert (MedicAlert Foundation, Turlock, CA) or similar warning bracelets or chains

- Avoid β-adrenergic blockers, angiotensin-converting enzyme inhibitors, monoamine oxidase inhibitors, and tricyclic antidepressants, if possible

- Where appropriate, use specific preventive strategies, including pharmacologic prophylaxis, provocative dose challenge, and desensitization

Adapted from Kemp SF. Office approach to anaphylaxis: sooner better than later. Am J Med 2007;120:667.

All individuals at risk for anaphylaxis should carry and know how to self-administer epinephrine. Because the potential benefit of epinephrine outweighs the risk of untreated anaphylaxis, patients should be strongly encouraged to self-administer epinephrine in any case of doubt.[19,21] Data are limited concerning the frequency with which 2 or more doses of epinephrine are needed to treat anaphylaxis (reports range from 16%–36%), and multiple cofactors may be involved.[19]

Demonstration of proper self-administration technique with a placebo trainer autoinjector is strongly recommended for patients and their family members, but many receive improper or no instructions.[19] Patients should promptly seek precautionary medical attention after self-administration of epinephrine. **Table 2** lists the single-dose epinephrine autoinjectors commercially available in North America.

The agent responsible for anaphylaxis in an individual must be identified, whenever possible, and instructions provided on how to minimize future exposure. The relative and relevant benefits and risks of certain medications (eg, angiotensin-converting enzyme inhibitors, β-blockers, monoamine oxidase inhibitors, and some tricyclic antidepressants) should be discussed, where applicable, with patients and their health care professionals and these medications should be discontinued if feasible.[2,12,15]

Patients with food-triggered anaphylaxis should scrutinize food labels and mitigate risk of ingesting food cross-contaminated during preparation. Accidental ingestion of peanuts and tree nuts is common.[21] Education is of paramount importance, and Food Allergy Research & Education (FARE; 800–929-4040; www.foodallergy.org) is a helpful nonprofit resource for many food-allergic individuals.

Specific immunoglobulin E (IgE) skin testing may help ascertain the potential for anaphylaxis in some circumstances (eg, allergy to β-lactam antibiotics or to protein excipients of certain vaccines). However, the immunochemistry of most drugs and biologic agents is not well defined.

Table 2
Single-dose epinephrine autoinjectors commercially available in North America

Name of Device	Manufacturer	Dose Injected IM in the Anterolateral Thigh
Adrenaclick[a]	Amedra Pharmaceuticals, Horsham, PA	Adults, 0.3 mg/0.3 mL Child ≥30 kg, 0.3 mg/0.3 mL Child <30 kg, 0.15 mg/0.15 mL
Allerject	Sanofi Canada, Laval, Quebec	Adults, 0.3 mg/0.3 mL Child ≥30 kg, 0.3 mg/0.3 mL Child <30 kg, 0.15 mg/0.15 mL
Auvi-Q	Sanofi US, Bridgewater, NJ	Adults, 0.3 mg/0.3 mL Child ≥30 kg, 0.3 mg/0.3 mL Child <30 kg, 0.15 mg/0.15 mL
EpiPen	Mylan Specialty US (Basking Ridge, NJ); also sublicensed through Pfizer Canada	Adults, 0.3 mg/0.3 mL IM Child ≥30 kg, 0.3 mg/0.3 mL
EpiPen Jr	—	Child <30 kg, 0.15 mg/0.3 mL

Adrenaclick and EpiPen/EpiPen Jr. are penlike devices with written instructions on each syringe barrel.
The Auvi-Q/Allerject is approximately the size of a credit card and features blinking lights at the needle end and a voice recording that guides the user throughout administration.
[a] Counterpart is not available in Canada.

Situations may arise in which it is necessary to administer a medication that previously caused anaphylaxis. Numerous protocols are available to assist in decreasing the risk of severe adverse reactions. These desensitization protocols should be conducted in clinical settings only where anaphylaxis, if it occurs, can be properly managed. Techniques used in these protocols include antihistamine and glucocorticoid prophylaxis to prevent or reduce the severity of IgE-independent reactions (eg, radiographic contrast media); administration of incremental doses of medication gradually over several hours (eg, short-term desensitization to penicillin, carboplatin); or the highly effective, long-term risk reduction with venom immunotherapy for insect sting anaphylaxis. Therapeutic preparations of anti-IgE monoclonal antibodies (omalizumab) may mitigate risk in some scenarios (eg, frequent idiopathic anaphylaxis), but more data are needed.[15]

SUMMARY

Education, avoidance, and prevention are critically important because some anaphylactic reactions are so severe that fatalities occur despite rapid recognition and treatment. Allergist-immunologists can provide comprehensive professional assistance. The treatment of choice for anaphylaxis is intramuscular epinephrine. Improving the evidence base for various treatment and preventive modalities through controlled trials may further help minimize fatalities from anaphylaxis.

REFERENCES

1. Khan BQ, Kemp SF. Pathophysiology of anaphylaxis. Curr Opin Allergy Clin Immunol 2011;11:319–25.
2. Brown SGA, Kemp SF, Lieberman PL. Anaphylaxis. In: Adkinson NF Jr, Bochner BS, Burks AW, et al, editors. Middleton's allergy: principles and practice. 8th edition. Philadelphia: Elsevier Saunders; 2014. p. 1237–59.
3. Sampson HA, Muñoz-Furlong A, Campbell RL, et al. Second symposium on the definition and management of anaphylaxis: summary report—second National Institute of Allergy and Infectious Disease/Food Allergy and Anaphylaxis Network symposium. J Allergy Clin Immunol 2006;117:391–7.
4. Campbell RL, Hagan JB, Manivannan V, et al. Evaluation of National Institute of Allergy and Infectious Diseases/Food Allergy and Anaphylaxis Network criteria for the diagnosis of anaphylaxis in emergency department patients. J Allergy Clin Immunol 2012;129:748–52.
5. Wood RA, Camargo CA Jr, Lieberman P, et al. Anaphylaxis in America: the prevalence and characteristics of anaphylaxis in the United States. J Allergy Clin Immunol 2014;133:461–7.
6. Tole JW, Lieberman P. Biphasic anaphylaxis: review of incidence, clinical predictors, and observation recommendations. Immunol Allergy Clin North Am 2007;27:309–26.
7. Kemp SF. The post-anaphylaxis dilemma: how long is long enough to observe a patient after resolution of symptoms? Curr Allergy Asthma Rep 2008;8:45–8.
8. Sheikh A, Shehata YA, Brown SGA, et al. Adrenaline for the treatment of anaphylaxis: Cochrane Systematic Review. Allergy 2009;64:204–12.
9. Sheikh A, Ten Broek V, Brown SGA, et al. H1-antihistamines for the treatment of anaphylaxis: Cochrane Systematic Review. Allergy 2007;62:830–7.
10. Nurmatov UB, Rhatigan E, Simons FER, et al. H2-antihistamines for the treatment of anaphylaxis with and without shock: a systematic review. Ann Allergy Asthma Immunol 2014;112:126–31.

11. Dhami S, Panesar SS, Roberts G, et al. Management of anaphylaxis: a systematic review. Allergy 2014;69:168–75.
12. Lieberman P, Nicklas RA, Oppenheimer J, et al. The diagnosis and management of anaphylaxis practice parameter: 2010 update. J Allergy Clin Immunol 2010; 126:477–80.e1–42.
13. VandenHoek TL, Morrison LJ, Shuster M, et al. Part 12: cardiac arrest in special situations: 2010 American Heart Association guidelines for cardiopulmonary resuscitation and emergency cardiovascular care. Circulation 2010; 122(Suppl 3):S829–61.
14. Soar J, Perkins JD, Abbas G, et al. European Resuscitation Council guidelines for resuscitation 2010 section 8. Cardiac arrest in special circumstances: electrolyte abnormalities, poisoning, drowning, accidental hypothermia, hyperthermia, asthma, anaphylaxis, cardiac surgery, trauma, pregnancy, electrocution. Resuscitation 2010;81:1400–33.
15. Simons FER, Ardusso LRF, Bilò MB, et al. World Allergy Organization guidelines for the assessment and management of anaphylaxis. J Allergy Clin Immunol 2011;127:587–93.e1–22.
16. Clark S, Bock SA, Gaeta TH, et al. Multicenter study of emergency department visits for food allergies. J Allergy Clin Immunol 2004;113:347–52.
17. Haymore BR, Carr WW, Frank WT. Anaphylaxis and epinephrine prescribing patterns in a military hospital: underutilization of the intramuscular route. Allergy Asthma Proc 2005;26:361–5.
18. Beyer K, Eckermann O, Hompes S, et al. Anaphylaxis in an emergency setting—elicitors, therapy and incidence of severe allergic reactions. Allergy 2012;67: 1451–6.
19. Kemp SF, Lockey RF, Simons FER. Epinephrine: the drug of choice for anaphylaxis. A statement of the World Allergy Organization. Allergy 2008;63:1061–70.
20. Simons FER, Ardusso LRF, Dimov V, et al. World Allergy Organization anaphylaxis guidelines: 2013 update of the evidence base. Int Arch Allergy Immunol 2013; 162:193–204.
21. NIAID-Sponsored Expert Panel. Guidelines for the diagnosis and management of food allergy in the United States: report of the NIAID-sponsored expert panel. J Allergy Clin Immunol 2010;126(Suppl 6):S1–58.
22. Cox L, Nelson H, Lockey R, et al. Allergen immunotherapy: a practice parameter third update. J Allergy Clin Immunol 2011;127:S1–55.
23. Westfall TC, Westfall DP. Adrenergic agonists and antagonists. In: Brunton LL, Chabner BA, Knollman BC, editors. Goodman and Gilman's the pharmacological basis of therapeutics. 12th edition. New York: Access Medicine from McGraw-Hill; 2011. Chapter 12.
24. Pumphrey R. Anaphylaxis: can we tell who is at risk of a fatal reaction? Curr Opin Allergy Clin Immunol 2004;4:285–90.
25. Simons FER. Pharmacologic treatment of anaphylaxis: can the evidence base be strengthened? Curr Opin Allergy Clin Immunol 2010;10:384–93.
26. Simons FER, Ardusso LRF, Bilò MB, et al. 2012 Update: World Allergy Organization guidelines for the assessment and management of anaphylaxis. Curr Opin Allergy Clin Immunol 2012;12:389–99.
27. Fisher MM. Clinical observations on the pathophysiology and treatment of anaphylactic cardiovascular collapse. Anaesth Intensive Care 1986;14: 17–21.
28. Pumphrey RS. Fatal posture in anaphylactic shock. J Allergy Clin Immunol 2003; 112:451–2.

29. Caroline NL. Emergency care in the streets. 2nd edition. Boston: Little, Brown; 1983. p. 57–98.
30. Kemp AM, Kemp SF. Pharmacotherapy in refractory anaphylaxis: when intramuscular epinephrine fails. Curr Opin Allergy Clin Immunol 2014;14:371–8.
31. McIntyre LA, Hebert PC, Fergusson D, et al. A survey of Canadian intensivists' resuscitation practices in early septic shock. Crit Care 2007;11:R74.
32. Takil A, Eti Z, Irmak P, et al. Early postoperative respiratory acidosis after large intravascular volume infusion of lactated Ringer's solution during major spine surgery. Anesth Analg 2002;95:294–8.
33. Neumar RW, Otto CW, Link MS, et al. Part 8: adult advanced cardiovascular life support: 2010 American Heart Association guidelines for cardiopulmonary resuscitation and emergency cardiovascular care. Circulation 2010;122(Suppl 3):S729–67.
34. Brown SGA, Blackman KE, Stenlake V, et al. Insect sting anaphylaxis: prospective evaluation of treatment with intravenous adrenaline and volume resuscitation. Emerg Med J 2004;21:149–54.
35. Sheikh A. Glucocorticosteroids for the treatment and prevention of anaphylaxis. Curr Opin Allergy Clin Immunol 2013;13:263–7.
36. Havel C, Arrich J, Losert H, et al. Vasopressors for hypotensive shock. Cochrane Database Syst Rev 2011;(5):CD003709.
37. Thomas M, Crawford I. Best evidence topic report. Glucagon infusion in refractory anaphylactic shock in patients on beta-blockers. Emerg Med J 2005; 22:272–3.
38. Skidgel RA, Kaplan AP, Erdös EG. Histamine, bradykinin, and their antagonists. In: Brunton LL, Chabner BA, Knollman BC, editors. Goodman and Gilman's the pharmacological basis of therapeutics. 12th edition. New York: Access Medicine from McGraw-Hill; 2011. Chapter 32.
39. Simons FE. Advances in H1-antihistamines. N Engl J Med 2004;351:2203–17.
40. Ellis BC, Brown SGA. Parenteral antihistamines cause hypotension in anaphylaxis. Emerg Med Australas 2013;25:92–3.
41. Schimmer BP, Funder JW. ACTH, adrenal steroids, and pharmacology of the adrenal cortex. In: Brunton LL, Chabner BA, Knollman BC, editors. Goodman and Gilman's the pharmacological basis of therapeutics. 12th edition. New York: Access Medicine from McGraw-Hill; 2011. Chapter 42.
42. Evora PR, Simon MR. Role of nitric oxide production in anaphylaxis and its relevance for the treatment of anaphylactic hypotension with methylene blue. Ann Allergy Asthma Immunol 2007;99:306–13.
43. Del Duca D, Sheth SS, Clarke AE, et al. Use of methylene blue for catecholamine-refractory vasoplegia from protamine and aprotinin. Ann Thorac Surg 2009;87: 640–2.
44. Bauer CS, Vadas P, Kelly KJ. Methylene blue for the treatment of refractory anaphylaxis without hypotension. Am J Emerg Med 2013;31:264.e3–5.
45. Dewachter P, Castro S, Nicaise-Roland P, et al. Anaphylactic reaction after methylene blue-treated plasma transfusion. Br J Anaesth 2011;106:687–9.
46. Nubret K, Delhoume M, Orsel I, et al. Anaphylactic shock to fresh-frozen plasma inactivated with methylene blue. Transfusion 2011;51:125–8.
47. Scranton SE, Gonzalez ED, Waibel KH. Incidence and characteristics of biphasic reactions after immunotherapy. J Allergy Clin Immunol 2009;123:493–8.

Fatal and Near-fatal Anaphylaxis

Factors That Can Worsen or Contribute to Fatal Outcomes

Paul A. Greenberger, MD

KEYWORDS

- Anaphylaxis • Allergy • Fatalities • Cardiovascular • Histamine • Prostaglandin
- Leukotriene

KEY POINTS

- Anaphylaxis implies a risk of death even in patients whose prior episodes have been considered trivial and easily managed.
- Anaphylaxis occurs in all age groups, from infants to the elderly, but most deaths occur in adults.
- Atopy is a risk factor for most types of anaphylaxis.
- There are no absolute contraindications to self-injectable epinephrine, and epinephrine can be administered for anaphylaxis to elderly patients or to those receiving beta-adrenergic blockers.

INTRODUCTION

Anaphylaxis is a medical emergency that implies a risk of death. Most cases of fatal or near-fatal anaphylaxis are characterized by abrupt-onset, progressively more severe symptoms, and short duration of time from exposure to the onset of symptoms. It has been reported that half or more of fatalities occur within 60 minutes of the onset of anaphylaxis.[1–6] Although full doses of medications, such as penicillins or neuromuscular blocking agents, may have been administered by the time signs or symptoms of anaphylaxis appear, severe symptoms can occur within a minute of administering intravenous medication and a single bite of a food can be associated with fatal or near-fatal anaphylaxis.[2,7–9] Anaphylactic deaths have occurred even

Supported by the Ernest S. Bazley Trust to Northwestern Memorial Hospital and Northwestern University.
Division of Allergy-Immunology, Department of Medicine, Northwestern University Feinberg School of Medicine, 211 East Ontario Street, #1000, Chicago, IL 60611, USA
E-mail address: p-greenberger@northwestern.edu

Immunol Allergy Clin N Am 35 (2015) 375–386
http://dx.doi.org/10.1016/j.iac.2015.01.001   **immunology.theclinics.com**
0889-8561/15/$ – see front matter © 2015 Elsevier Inc. All rights reserved.

when the bite of food was spat out and not swallowed or aspirated,[7] and with just a test dose of 1 to 2 mL of radiographic contrast material.[10] Often, in fatalities, epinephrine was not immediately administered.[2,7,8]

PATHOPHYSIOLOGY OF FATAL AND NEAR-FATAL ANAPHYLAXIS

The prototype reaction is uniphasic, beginning within minutes or up to 2 to 3 hours after exposure to the cause; some reactions are biphasic, in which the immediate reaction seems to stop for at least 1 hour before returning; and some are protracted, in which the immediate reaction continues for hours or days. Cases of protracted anaphylaxis can last from 3 days to 3 weeks.[8]

Mast cell activation is one mechanism of anaphylaxis, and laboratory evidence of such is shown by an increased total serum tryptase concentration (>11.4 ng/mL) or increased urine histamine or N-methylhistamine concentration. Serum histamine measurement is not of practical use because of its short half-life. Preformed mediators within the mast cell include histamine, chymase, tryptase, carboxypeptidase, and cathepsin G. Intravenous infusions of histamine can cause pruritus, flushing, urticaria, chest tightness, and eventually a reduction in blood pressure.[11] However, other mediators are thought to contribute to an even greater extent in anaphylaxis. For example, newly synthesized mediators, including prostaglandin D2, leukotriene D4, and platelet-activating factor are released, all of which can dilate blood vessels and potently contract smooth muscle. Kinins, which can cause relaxation of smooth muscle and increased capillary permeability, are also generated during anaphylaxis and likely contribute to acute angioedema, such as massive tongue swelling or hypotensive shock. It remains unclear to what extent tryptase contributes to the pathophysiologic changes of anaphylaxis.

In fatal or near-fatal anaphylaxis, physiologic changes such as the following may be found: (1) hypotensive (distributive) shock from reduced total peripheral resistance and permeable capillaries, with loss of up to 35% of intravascular volume[12]; (2) massive angioedema of the tongue, oropharynx, or larynx; (3) cardiac arrhythmias, such as atrial or ventricular fibrillation with or without myocardial infarction[6,9,13]; and (4) acute severe bronchoconstriction. It remains uncertain why the shock organ varies in different individuals in fatal and near-fatal anaphylaxis but it seems that, in patients with asthma, the lung is commonly the shock organ[7,8] and often contributes to death or respiratory failure.

During intraoperative anaphylaxis occurring in patients with cardiac catheters in place, there was a transient increase of the pulmonary artery pressure, likely from bronchoconstriction, in association with a catastrophic reduction in peripheral resistance.[12] These findings were identified in patients with underlying cardiac disease resulting in greatly reduced blood volume reaching the left ventricle to support the blood pressure or cardiac output. Even in the absence of cardiac disease, patients can present with sudden-onset cardiovascular collapse, myocardial infarction, or ventricular fibrillation.[13] Cardiac ischemia during anaphylaxis can result from activation of mast cells that are located in the interstitium and adventitia of the larger coronary arteries.[14]

Acute severe bronchoconstriction may necessitate ventilatory support because patients can present with respiratory failure with arterial blood gases with pH of 6.95 to 7.05 and Pco_2 greater than 90 mm Hg. In this setting, it may be difficult to deliver an effective tidal volume to the patient without using high and potentially dangerous inspiratory pressures. This emergency has led to use of extracorporeal membrane oxygenation.[15]

PATHOLOGY AND LABORATORY FINDINGS

The findings from autopsy examinations of fatal anaphylaxis are listed in **Box 1**. Obstructing angioedema of the upper airway can cause death from asphyxiation. Some patients experience acute myocardial infarction from hypotension or cardiac arrest during fatal or near-fatal anaphylaxis. Patients may not present with urticaria, especially if hypotensive. Although infrequent in patients presenting with unexplained shock, the emergence of urticaria as the patient is being resuscitated can raise the possibility that anaphylaxis has occurred. This scenario can be observed in patients who have been stung by an insect or who have idiopathic anaphylaxis.[13] First responders can help restore the blood pressure and increase cardiac output to peripheral tissues, allowing urticarial lesions to appear.

Results of laboratory investigations in anaphylaxis include:

- The cutoff for serum tryptase concentrations for fatal anaphylaxis is greater than or equal to 44.3 ng/mL.[16,17] Postmortem serum tryptase concentrations can be greater than 11.4 ng/mL when patients die from nonanaphylactic conditions, including asphyxia (from smothering, suicide, or external compression of the chest), assault, sudden infant death syndrome, sudden cardiac death, acute aortic dissection, heroin injection, and trauma such as from a motor vehicle accident.[16,17] A concentration greater than or equal to 44.3 ng/mL best differentiates between fatal anaphylaxis and deaths from other causes. There may be some false-negatives in cases of fatal anaphylaxis, such as when the serum tryptase concentration is increased but lower than the cutoff (18 and 37 ng/mL)[10] or in the normal range (such as in food allergy[8,18]). However, the serum tryptase concentration can be sharply increased and greater than or equal to 44.3 ng/mL in fatalities from food-induced anaphylaxis.[18]

- Increased serum immunoglobulin E (IgE) antibodies to foods and stinging or biting insects provide supportive information in exploring causes of fatal anaphylaxis.[18] The results of such determinations can be useful, especially when the serum tryptase concentration is modestly increased (12 ng/mL for fatal soybean-induced anaphylaxis and 17 ng/mL for fatal codfish-induced anaphylaxis).[18] Postmortem serum should be stored frozen at −20°C to preserve IgE antibodies and tryptase. Serum tryptase may still have 50% of its concentration after storage at room temperature for 4 days.[18]

- The normal range for histamine in whole blood in living subjects is less than 0.3 ng/mL.[19] In one report, concentrations from cases of fatal anaphylaxis

---

Box 1
Pathologic findings in fatal anaphylaxis

Angioedema	Massive (obstructing) edema of tongue, lips, larynx, supraglottic area, or epiglottis
Hyperinflation of the lungs	Resembles emphysematous changes
Tracheobronchial secretions	
Mucus plugging of airways	
Congestion	Viscera and lungs (sometimes with pulmonary edema)
Cyanosis	Face and body
Coronary atherosclerosis	Coincidental finding in some patients
Cerebral hypoxia	Global cerebral ischemia
Cutaneous urticaria	
Cutaneous angioedema	
No specific findings	Presumed sudden, severe cardiovascular collapse

were 37.5, 9.0, and 23.2 ng/mL, compared with controls from nonanaphylactic deaths, such as sudden cardiac death, ranging from 5.0 to 22 ng/mL.[19] Thus, there is modest evidence for demonstration of increased blood histamine level in fatal anaphylaxis, but, in terms of utility, all 3 cases of anaphylactic death had serum tryptase concentrations greater than or equal to 45 ng/mL, therefore tryptase concentrations are more feasible with histamine as an adjunct if needed.

- The normal range for diamine oxidase, one of 2 enzymes that degrade histamine (the other being histamine-N-methyltransferase), is 10 to 30 IU/mL.[19] There was no meaningful difference between concentrations of diamine oxidase in 3 cases of fatal anaphylaxis compared with controls.[19] These preliminary results do not support the notion that there might be a deficiency of diamine oxidase in fatal anaphylaxis.
- Serum concentrations of platelet-activating factor are increased compared with controls and correlate directly with the severity of anaphylaxis.[20] There is an inverse correlation between platelet-activating factor acetylhydrolase and severity of anaphylaxis. These findings suggest that there may be insufficient degradation of platelet-activating factor in severe or fatal anaphylaxis.[20]
- In the setting of non-IgE, non–FcεRI-associated anaphylaxis from oversulfated chondroitin sulfate (OSCS) adulterated heparin, the OSCS caused robust in vitro increases in the levels of kallikrein and anaphylatoxins C5a and C3a from plasma.[21,22]

FACTORS OR CIRCUMSTANCES ASSOCIATED WITH FATAL OR NEAR-FATAL ANAPHYLAXIS

Various factors that can contribute to a fatal or near-fatal anaphylactic reaction have been identified (**Box 2**). For example, in adults presenting with anaphylaxis, the use of antihypertensive medications (in aggregate) was associated with involvement of 3 or more organ systems and risk of hospitalization.[23] The risk of hospitalization was associated with the severity of anaphylaxis as determined by the presence of at least 1 of the following severity markers: syncope, hypoxia, hypotension, and more than 1 injection of epinephrine.[23]

The following discussion considers settings, factors, or circumstances associated with fatal or near-fatal anaphylaxis.

Box 2
Factors or circumstances associated with near-fatal or fatal anaphylaxis

Accidents and mishaps

Adulterated products

Age

Allergens

Atopy

Comorbidities

Munchausen syndrome–contrived anaphylaxis

Patient factors

Route of administration

Treatment-related issues

Accidents and Mishaps

Examples include:

1. Patients confusing medications or nonprescription products. In one case this resulted in ingestion of amoxicillin instead of ascorbic acid.[9]
2. Systems errors. Patients receive a medication to which they are known to be allergic, despite the medical record clearly listing the allergy; or the allergy is listed but the physician or health care professional minimizes the significance of the reaction; or the patient's allergy is not entered into the medical record.
3. Administrative errors in identification of the patient or of the dosage of medication or allergen immunotherapy to be administered.
4. Anaphylaxis in remote areas where first aid is delayed or not likely.
5. Self-injectable epinephrine is not available or not used promptly.
6. Incorrect assumptions about foods, such as assuming that certain peanut-free foods are devoid of allergen, or when the patient or responsible party assumes that the patient is now immune (nonsusceptible) to the risk of anaphylaxis and eats the allergenic food.

Adulterated Products

There may be intentional adulteration of medications (as in the use of OSCS in heparin) or foods (such as hazelnut oil substituted for extravirgin olive oil.) The allergenic risk in the latter example is when there is detectable hazelnut protein in hazelnut oil.[24,25] In general, refined oils have less protein content than partially refined oils, which have less protein than crude oils. Alternatively, there may be unintentional adulteration of an initially safe food product, such as when a cook adds a tablespoon of peanut butter to a gallon of peanut oil so that, when prepared, the tortillas fold, adhere, and taste better.

Age

Although deaths or nearly fatal anaphylaxis occur in children and adolescents,[7,8] the literature shows that the preponderance of fatalities occur in adults.[1–6,12,13,26] Near-fatal anaphylaxis can occur in persons of any age, from infants to the geriatric population. Adolescents may not make safe decisions regarding what to eat. They may not successfully self-inject epinephrine when indicated or may not carry the epinephrine because of negative peer pressure. Alternatively, they may be subject to bullying and having the known food allergen intentionally placed into their lunches at school.[27,28] Adults may be reluctant to self-inject epinephrine because previous episodes of anaphylaxis have been tolerated after ingestion of 200 mg of diphenhydramine or hydroxyzine.

Another aspect of age is the intrinsic reactivity from allergic reactions that can increase with age. In a review of children and adolescents who were known to have had positive double-blind, placebo-controlled food challenges, the eliciting dose of the food declined as children aged.[29] Regarding peanut allergy, the median dose for a positive challenge was 790 mg in children less than 5 years of age, 310 mg in children 5 to 10 years of age, and just 70 mg in children 11 years and older.[29] These findings were unaffected by the presence of asthma.

Allergens

The potency of allergens is variable, and attempts have been made to determine the lowest dose of allergens that cause an observable adverse effect. If the highest dose tolerated is known, this could affect product manufacturing and labeling. This information would be valuable for policy making because fatalities or near-fatal anaphylaxis have occurred after single bites of peanuts, tree nuts, seeds, and other foods.[7–9]

Roasted peanuts are more allergenic than boiled peanuts.[30–32] There are 11 well-characterized allergens in peanut, and heating increases the binding of *Ara h* 1 and *Ara h* 2 to IgE antibodies.[30] Furthermore, heated *Ara h* 2 adsorbed to human intestinal epithelial cells to a greater extent, which could result in enhanced signaling and subsequent immunoreactivity.[30]

The use of component-resolved immunoassays for diagnosis of food allergies may help elucidate the differential susceptibilities of allergic patients to various foods. For example, shrimp tropomyosin (*Pen a* 1) is considered the major allergen in patients with shrimp allergy, but other allergens are being recognized.[33] In sera from 15 patients with shrimp-induced anaphylaxis, just 7 showed anti-*Pen a* 1 IgE antibodies. As experience is gained with component-resolved immunoassays, it is hoped that risk assessment will be improved, ideally into true anaphylaxis-prone, urticaria-prone, and oral allergy syndrome–prone categories.

The allergen may not be a food but a contaminant in the food, such as wheat flour contaminated by dust or storage mite ingested by a person allergic to dust mites.[34,35] Contamination of foods such as pancakes, beignets, grits, polenta, pizza dough, and mackerel or bonito covered in flour has been described.[34] There are heat-resistant and heat-labile allergens in mites, but it is the heat-resistant allergens that seem to cause anaphylaxis, and can be near fatal (acute respiratory failure) or fatal.[34,35] This form of anaphylaxis is preventable with proper storage of flour.

There is a single case report of fatal anaphylaxis after consumption of presumably 2 mold-contaminated pancakes.[36] A 19-year-old man with asthma and allergies, who was not apparently allergic to dust or eggs, died after eating pancakes that had been prepared with flour that had been opened previously and had a use-by date that had expired 2 years earlier. A variety of fungi were identified in the pancake mix, including *Aspergillus flavus* and *Aspergillus niger*, *Penicillium* species, *Fusarium* species, and *Mucor*.[36] Two friends of the deceased stopped eating the pancakes because the pancakes tasted like rubbing alcohol.[36] It is not known whether the anaphylaxis was attributable to mites instead of fungi, and mites were not tested for in the report.

Atopy

Atopy is a risk factor for most, but not all, causes of anaphylaxis. This information is presented in **Table 1**.

Comorbidities

Comorbidities can contribute to the risk of an unfavorable outcome from anaphylaxis and have been identified in 22 of 25 fatal cases in which the mean age of patients was 59 years.[2] Postmortem findings often include coexisting evidence of asthma, emphysema, or preexisting cardiovascular disease, such as coronary or aortic atherosclerosis, myocardial ischemia, or valvular heart disease.

Asthma, especially if severe, has been recognized as a risk factor for anaphylaxis.[37,38] After controlling for age, sex, race/ethnicity, co morbidities, and allergen immunotherapy, there was a 5.2-fold increased incidence of anaphylactic shock in patients with asthma.[38]

Patients with indolent systemic mastocytosis are known to be susceptible to systemic reactions from Hymenoptera stings. The finding of an increased serum tryptase concentration or lesions of urticaria pigmentosa in a patient with venom

Table 1 Effect of atopy on types of anaphylaxis	
Atopy Is a Risk Factor	**Atopy Is Not a Risk Factor**
Asthma (especially if persistent severe)	Penicillin
Exercise-induced anaphylaxis	Neuromuscular blocking agents
Food	Insulin
Idiopathic anaphylaxis	
Hymenoptera	
Latex	
Radiographic contrast media	

anaphylaxis may lead to the diagnosis of indolent systemic mastocytosis in previously undiagnosed patients.

By definition, idiopathic anaphylaxis (IA) implies a risk of death or severe anaphylaxis.[13,39–41] Use of empiric prednisone compared with H1 antihistamines alone has been associated with favorable outcomes, including reduced frequency of episodes and severity of this condition.[40,41] IA-Frequent means that there have been 6 episodes of anaphylaxis in the past 12 months or 2 within the past 2 months. IA-Infrequent means that there have been 5 or fewer episodes of anaphylaxis in the past 12 months.

As noted earlier, patients receiving antihypertensive medications (taken in aggregate) are at increased risk of anaphylaxis.[23] β-Blockers, angiotensin-converting enzyme inhibitors, and diuretics analyzed individually did not correlate with syncope, hypotension, or hypoxia.[23] Bradykinin, which causes vasodilatation and angioedema, is degraded primarily by angiotensin-converting enzyme. It has been reported that patients with peanut and tree allergy who had lower concentrations of serum angiotensin-converting enzyme had more severe pharyngeal edema.[42]

Beta-adrenergic blocking agents may or may not potentiate the severity or increase the incidence of anaphylaxis. For example, in a prospective study of patients undergoing cardiac angiography, there was not an increased risk of anaphylaxis during radiographic contrast material infusions in patients receiving beta-adrenergic blockers,[43] although this has been reported from a retrospective, case control study.[44] Nor was there an increased risk of anaphylaxis in patients undergoing allergen immunotherapy.[45] Nevertheless, the use of beta-adrenergic blockers may identify patients with underlying cardiovascular disease (but it should be remembered that epinephrine is not contraindicated in patients taking these medications because of the potential for coronary ischemia or hypertension). Although there have been concerns that systemically administered epinephrine might cause exaggerated alpha-adrenergic effects when administered to patients receiving beta-adrenergic blockers during treatment of anaphylaxis, it is more likely that the anaphylactic shock will be difficult to reverse and that additional doses of epinephrine may be required along with other measures of resuscitation.

The concomitant use of moderate to high doses of tricyclic antidepressants may potentiate the effects of epinephrine, but any such drug-drug interactions are expected to be more severe in the setting of a monoamine oxidase inhibitor or cocaine.

Munchausen Syndrome–contrived Anaphylaxis

Munchausen stridor is nonorganic laryngeal obstruction in which the perpetrator produces loud, frightening, stridorous sounds, often resulting in emergency intubation.[46,47] Some nonintubated patients are treated with intravenous epinephrine for ongoing stridor that perplexes inexperienced physicians. In contrast, Munchausen anaphylaxis is true anaphylaxis.[48,49] For example, a patient with purported Hymenoptera anaphylaxis provoked anaphylactic signs and symptoms from her established aspirin hypersensitivity by surreptitious ingestion of aspirin to convince others that Hymenoptera stings were the cause.[48] Patients with Munchausen syndrome can provoke severe or potentially fatal factitious disease, including anaphylaxis, and are often resistant to professional advice or psychiatric treatment because the underlying disorder results in secondary gain.

Patient Factors

Patients who have experienced anaphylaxis can have impaired quality of life for multiple reasons, including:

1. Anxiety, panic, hypochondriasis, or depression about future episodes and loss of control of their health.
2. Uncertainty as to the cause of the anaphylaxis or how to prevent future episodes.
3. Lack of a management plan, including whether, when, and how to self-administer epinephrine.
4. Therapeutic nihilism that meaningful interventions from health care professionals are available. In patients with IA, in addition to concurrent pharmacotherapy directed at IA, psychiatric consultation and therapy can be effective in patients who become depressed about anaphylaxis, as has been shown in patients with IA-F. Fatalities have been described in patients with IA when empiric treatment has not been undertaken by patients.[39]

When patients minimize or deny the potential severity of future episodes of anaphylaxis, life-threatening conditions can occur. For example, a 19-year-old college student with peanut allergy while in a bar accepted a dare to eat 1 peanut. Shortly thereafter, he experienced life-threatening respiratory distress and required intubation, with a Pco_2 of more than 90 mm Hg and pH less than 7.0. The patient survived but did not want to accept responsibility for his unwise and dangerous intentional ingestion of a peanut.

Another example is that of patients who minimize or deny the risks of future anaphylactic episodes from Hymenoptera stings or are unaware of an immunomodulatory treatment, and do not receive the salutary protective benefits of venom immunotherapy.

Route of Administration

Fatal and severe to near-fatal anaphylaxis can occur with any route of administration (intravenous, intra-arterial, intraarticular, oral, contact, inhalational, kissing, and penile-vaginal sexual intercourse). The median time to shock, respiratory arrest, or cardiac arrest from a series of 20 fatal episodes of anaphylaxis was as follows: iatrogenic (systemically administered) reactions, 5 minutes; venom stings, 15 minutes; and foods, 30 minutes.[26] In a series of 25 cases of fatal anaphylaxis, the anaphylactic event started within 30 minutes of exposure in 20 of 25 cases, with death in 60 minutes in 13 of 25 cases.[2] These findings support the belief that the more rapid the reaction following exposure to the antigen, the worse the anaphylaxis may be.

Treatment-related Issues

In addition to delays in the diagnosis of anaphylactic shock and initiation of treatment with epinephrine and, when feasible, intravenous fluids, the attempted first aid of patients while in the sitting and upright positions has been reported as being associated with sudden demise.[50] Specifically, the abrupt change in posture (from seated or lying down to standing, or from lying in bed to sitting in a chair) has been associated with sudden death from anaphylaxis.[50] The loss of intravascular volume resulting in little filling pressure into the right ventricle with reduced cardiac output has led to the term empty ventricle syndrome.[50] The recommendation is that, when patients are in anaphylactic shock, they should be treated in the supine position (as tolerated, depending on level of dyspnea), with legs elevated to try to make the inferior vena cava the most dependent vessel. Also, antishock trousers can be used for this purpose.[50]

SUMMARY

Most episodes of anaphylaxis do not result in a fatality and the goal of treatment must be to prevent deaths and future reactions. A high-risk situation may be one in which mitigating factors are not recognized or opportunities for improvement are over-looked, and this applies to anaphylaxis. Therefore, in any patient with anaphylaxis, an allergy-immunology consultation is indicated to help confirm or rule out allergens, to teach about avoidance as well as risks, to possibly reduce risk (IA, venom allergy), and for optimal treatment of anaphylaxis.[51] For patients who have experienced anaphylaxis from Hymenoptera stings or fire ant bites, immunotherapy is highly effective to reduce the risk of future stings or bites. Empiric treatment of patients with frequent episodes of idiopathic anaphylaxis with prednisone and H1 antihista-mines can help modify the natural history of this condition by reducing the frequency and severity of episodes, and empiric treatment with H1 antihistamines and on-demand epinephrine is ineffective for acute episodes in most patients with IA-I. Self-injectable epinephrine remains indicated, and patients should be taught whether, when, and how to administer it as part of an individualized action plan.[51,52]

REFERENCES

1. Delage C, Irey NS. Anaphylactic deaths: a clinicopathologic study of 43 cases. J Forensic Sci 1972;17:525–40.
2. Pumphrey RS, Roberts IS. Postmortem findings after fatal anaphylactic reactions. J Clin Pathol 2000;53:273–6.
3. Greenberger PA, Rotskoff BD, Lifschultz B. Fatal anaphylaxis: postmortem findings and associated comorbid diseases. Ann Allergy Asthma Immunol 2007;98:252–7.
4. Riches KJ, Gillis D, James JA. An autopsy approach to bee sting-related deaths. Pathology 2002;34:257–62.
5. Low I, Stables S. Anaphylactic deaths in Auckland, New Zealand: a review of coronial autopsies from 1985 to 2005. Pathology 2006;38:328–32.
6. James LP, Austen KF. Fatal systemic anaphylaxis in man. N Engl J Med 1964;270: 597–603.
7. Bock SA, Munoz-Furlong A, Sampson HA. Fatalities due to anaphylactic reactions to foods. J Allergy Clin Immunol 2001;107:191–3.
8. Sampson HA, Mendelson L, Rosen JP. Fatal and near-fatal anaphylactic reactions to foods in children and adolescents. N Engl J Med 1992;327:380–4.
9. Golbert TM, Patterson R, Pruzansky JJ. Systemic allergic reactions to ingested antigens. J Allergy 1969;44:96–107.
10. Yamaguchi K, Katayama H, Takashima T, et al. Prediction of severe adverse reactions to ionic and nonionic contrast media in Japan: evaluation of pretesting. A report from the Japanese Committee on the Safety of Contrast Media. Radiology 1991;178:363–7.

11. Kaliner M, Sigler R, Summers R, et al. Effects of infused histamine: analysis of the effects of H-1 and H-2 histamine receptor antagonists on cardiovascular and pulmonary responses. J Allergy Clin Immunol 1981;68:365–71.

12. Fisher MM. Clinical observations on the pathophysiology and treatment of anaphylactic cardiovascular collapse. Anaesth Intensive Care 1986; 14:17–21.

13. Wong S, Greenberger PA, Patterson R. Nearly fatal idiopathic anaphylactic reaction resulting in cardiovascular collapse and myocardial infarction. Chest 1990;98:501–3.

14. Perskvist N, Edston E. Differential accumulation of pulmonary and cardiac mast cell-subsets and eosinophils between fatal anaphylaxis and asthma death: a postmortem comparative study. Forensic Sci Int 2007;169:43–9.

15. Lafforgue E, Sleth JC, Pluskwa F, et al. Successful extracorporeal resuscitation of a probable perioperative anaphylactic shock due to atracurium. Ann Fr Anesth Reanim 2005;24:551–5.

16. Edston E, Eriksson O, Van Hage M. Mast cell tryptase in postmortem serum—reference values and confounders. Int J Legal Med 2007;121:275–80.

17. Edston E, van Hage-Hamsten M. β-Tryptase measurements post-mortem in anaphylactic deaths and in controls. Forensic Sci Int 1998;93:135–42.

18. Yuninger JW, Nelson DR, Squillace DL, et al. Laboratory investigation of deaths due to anaphylaxis. J Forensic Sci 1991;36:857–65.

19. Mayer DE, Krauskopf A, Hemmer W, et al. Usefulness of post mortem determination of serum tryptase, histamine and diamine oxidase in the diagnosis of fatal anaphylaxis. Forensic Sci Int 2011;212:96–101.

20. Vadas P, Gold M, Perelman B, et al. Platelet-activating factor, PAF acetylhydrolase, and severe anaphylaxis. N Engl J Med 2008;358:28–35.

21. Blossum DB, Kallen AJ, Patel PR, et al. Outbreak of adverse reactions associated with contaminated heparin. N Engl J Med 2008;359:2674–84.

22. Kishimoto TK, Viswanathan K, Ganguly T, et al. Contaminated heparin associated with adverse clinical events and activation of the contact system. N Engl J Med 2008;358:2457–67.

23. Lee S, Hess EP, Nestler DM, et al. Antihypertensive medication use is associated with increased organ system involvement and hospitalization in emergency department patients with anaphylaxis. J Allergy Clin Immunol 2013;131:1103–8.

24. De Ceglie C, Calvano CD, Zambonin CG. Determination of hidden hazelnut oil proteins in extra virgin olive oil by cold acetone precipitation followed by in-solution tryptic digestion and MALDI-TOF-MS analysis. J Agric Food Chem 2014;62:9401–9.

25. Teuber SS, Brown RL, Haapanen LA. Allergenicity of gourmet nut oils processed by different methods. J Allergy Clin Immunol 1997;99:502–7.

26. Pumphrey RS. Lessons for management of anaphylaxis from a study of fatal reactions. Clin Exp Allergy 2000;30:1144–50.

27. Lieberman JA, Weiss C, Furlong TJ, et al. Bullying among pediatric patients with food allergy. Ann Allergy Asthma Immunol 2010;105:282–6.

28. Shemesh E, Annunziato RA, Ambrose MA, et al. Child and parental reports of bullying in a consecutive sample of children with food allergy. Pediatrics 2013; 131(1):e10–7.

29. van der Zee T, Dubois A, Kerkhof M, et al. The eliciting dose of peanut in double-blind, placebo-controlled food challenges decreases with increasing age and specific IgE level in children and young adults. J Allergy Clin Immunol 2011; 128:1031–6.

30. Starkl P, Krishnamurthy D, Szalai K, et al. Heating affects structure, enterocyte adsorption and signalling, as well as immunogenicity of the peanut allergen Ara h 2. Open Allergy J 2011;4:24–34.
31. Verma AK, Kumar S, Das M, et al. Impact of thermal processing on legume allergens. Plant Foods Hum Nutr 2012;67:430–41.
32. Vissers YM, Iwan M, Adel-Patient K, et al. Effect of roasting on the allergenicity of major peanut allergens Ara h 1 and Ara h 2/6: the necessity of degranulation assays. Clin Exp Allergy 2011;41:1631–42.
33. Asero R, Mistrello G, Amato S, et al. Shrimp allergy in Italian adults: a multicenter study showing a high prevalence of sensitivity to novel high molecular weight allergens. Int Arch Allergy Immunol 2012;157:3–10.
34. Sanchez-Borges M, Chacon RS, Capriles-Hulett A, et al. Anaphylaxis from ingestion of mites: pancake anaphylaxis. J Allergy Clin Immunol 2013; 131:31–5.
35. Edston E, van Hage-Hamstem M. Death in anaphylaxis in a man with house dust mite allergy. Int J Legal Med 2003;117:299–301.
36. Bennett AT, Collins KA. An unusual case of anaphylaxis: mold in pancake mix. Am J Forensic Med Pathol 2001;22:292–5.
37. Gonzalez-Perez A, Aponte Z, Vidaurre C, et al. Anaphylaxis epidemiology in patients with and patients without asthma: a United Kingdom database review. J Allergy Clin Immunol 2010;125:1098–104.
38. Iribarren C, Tolstykh IV, Miller MK, et al. Asthma and the prospective risk of anaphylactic shock and other allergy diagnoses in a large integrated health care delivery system. Ann Allergy Asthma Immunol 2010;104:371–7.
39. Patterson R, Clayton DE, Booth BH, et al. Fatal and near fatal idiopathic anaphylaxis. Allergy Proc 1995;16:103–8.
40. Ditto AM, Harris KE, Krasnick J, et al. Idiopathic anaphylaxis: a series of 335 cases. Ann Allergy Asthma Immunol 1996;77:285–91.
41. Wong S, Yarnold PR, Yango C, et al. Outcome of prophylactic therapy for idiopathic anaphylaxis. Ann Intern Med 1991;114:133–6.
42. Summers CW, Pumphrey RS, Woods CN, et al. Factors predicting anaphylaxis to peanuts and tree nuts in patients referred to a specialist center. J Allergy Clin Immunol 2008;121:632–8.
43. Greenberger PA, Meyers SN, Kramer BL, et al. Effects of beta-adrenergic and calcium antagonists on the development of anaphylactoid reactions from radiographic contrast media during cardiac angiography. J Allergy Clin Immunol 1987;80:698–702.
44. Lang DM, Alpern MB, Visintainer PF, et al. Elevated risk of anaphylactoid reaction from radiographic contrast media is associated with both beta-blocker exposure and cardiovascular disorders. Arch Intern Med 1993; 153:2033–40.
45. Hepner MJ, Ownby DR, Anderson JA, et al. Risk of systemic reactions in patients taking beta-blocker drugs receiving allergen immunotherapy injections. J Allergy Clin Immunol 1990;86:407–11.
46. Bahna SL, Oldham JL. Munchausen stridor—A strong false alarm of anaphylaxis. Allergy Asthma Immunol Res 2014;6(6):577–9.
47. Patterson R, Schatz M, Horton M. Munchausen's stridor: non-organic laryngeal obstruction. Clin Allergy 1974;4:307–10.
48. Hendrix S, Sale S, Zeiss CR, et al. Factitious Hymenoptera allergic emergency: a report of a new variant of Munchausen's syndrome. J Allergy Clin Immunol 1981; 67:8–13.

49. Lieberman P, Nicklas RA, Oppenheimer J, et al. The diagnosis and management of anaphylaxis practice parameter: 2010 update. J Allergy Clin Immunol 2010; 126:477–80.
50. Pumphrey RS. Fatal posture in anaphylactic shock. J Allergy Clin Immunol 2003; 112:451–2.
51. Lieberman PL. Recognition and first-line treatment of anaphylaxis. Am J Med 2014;127:S6–11.
52. Simons FE, Ardusso LR, Bilò MB, et al. International consensus on (ICON) anaphylaxis. World Allergy Organ J 2014;7(1):9 eCollection 2014.

Moving?

Make sure your subscription moves with you!

To notify us of your new address, find your **Clinics Account Number** (located on your mailing label above your name), and contact customer service at:

Email: journalscustomerservice-usa@elsevier.com

800-654-2452 (subscribers in the U.S. & Canada)
314-447-8871 (subscribers outside of the U.S. & Canada)

Fax number: 314-447-8029

Elsevier Health Sciences Division
Subscription Customer Service
3251 Riverport Lane
Maryland Heights, MO 63043

*To ensure uninterrupted delivery of your subscription, please notify us at least 4 weeks in advance of move.

Moving?

Make sure your subscription moves with you!

To notify us of your new address, find your Clinics Account Number (located on your mailing label above your name) and contact customer service at:

Email: journalscustomerservice-usa@elsevier.com

800-654-2452 (subscribers in the U.S. & Canada)
314-447-8871 (subscribers outside of the U.S. & Canada)

Fax number: 314-447-8029

Elsevier Health Sciences Division
Subscription Customer Service
3251 Riverport Lane
Maryland Heights, MO 63043

Printed and bound by CPI Group (UK) Ltd, Croydon, CR0 4YY

21/10/2024

01777267-0004